MW00467191

THE
SPANISH
MOLECULE

AND OTHER ADVENTURES IN ADDICTION PSYCHIATRY

DANIEL MIERLAK, MD, PHD

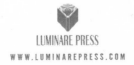

LUMINARE PRESS

WWW.LUMINAREPRESS.COM

AUTHOR'S NOTE

To protect the individuals involved in the following cases, names, dates, locations, and other details have been changed. It is important to note that no claim is made as to how substance use or psychiatric disorders ought to be treated, and none should be taken from the specific treatments mentioned in this volume.

THE SPANISH MOLECULE
And Other Adventures in Addiction Psychiatry

Printed in the United States of America

Cover Design by Claire Flint Last

Luminare Press
442 Charnelton St.
Eugene, OR 97401
www.luminarepress.com

LCCN: 2020922967
ISBN: 978-1-64388-525-4

For
Pamela, Victor, Elena, Harold, Dorothy,
Lindhoff, Richie, Evan, Andrei,
and unfortunate Lombardi

Out of the crooked timber of humanity,
no straight thing was ever made.

—EMMANUEL KANT

TABLE OF CONTENTS

FOREWORD

At the start of his career, psychiatrist and addiction specialist Daniel Mierlak had considered a more civilized calling in the seminar rooms and laboratories of academic science. He spent long days culturing chick neurons to chart the idiosyncrasies of a certain receptor. I imagine he had hoped to one day fashion a useful compound—the eponymous Spanish Molecule perhaps. But he decided to leave the relative tranquility of science for the grinding uncertainties of clinical practice. The young Dr. Mierlak, we must assume, craved adventure. And so he cast off the pipette and the electrode and girded himself with the crude tools available to the modern alienist: a scant apothecary drawer, reasonable common sense, and a strong stomach. He set forth, in Blake's words, to "walk in perilous paths," to try his hand at that marriage of heaven and hell that is clinical psychiatry. As the author demonstrates, ours is a discipline with one foot in miraculous twenty-first century neuroscience and the other still mired in conceptual opacity and wishful thinking. As an empiricist, with a deep understanding of the complexities of chick neurons, the author surely must have appreciated the pitfalls that awaited him in the messy realm of patient care.

But he pushed off from solid ground nonetheless. And so we are curious: how has this gone for you, Dr. Mierlak? From these tales one has to assume Dr. Mierlak cannot help shaking his head at the younger version of himself—the kid from Queens who naively saw romance in madhouse lore, hushed consulting rooms, and a downtown clientele. As the reader will learn, the astute Dr. Mierlak quickly acquires an important weapon in his battle against mental illness—the posture of therapeutic realism. Indeed, diminished expectations (of the doctor, of the patient, of the whole enterprise) emerges as a major theme throughout this collection. And so a protective skepticism, as well as nagging self-doubt, are Dr. Mierlak's constant companions as he struggles against the limits of a young science, the stubbornness of human misery, and the relentless fixity of mammalian behavior.

The trick of these tales is that, as we eavesdrop on Dr. Mierlak and his patients, we regret his foolhardy decision to forsake an honest living but are secretly pleased that he had the courage to run away and join the circus. And quite the high-wire act it turns out to be! Indeed the entire volume can be read as a tribute to the balancing act that clinical medicine often resembles: Dr. Mierlak realizes, despite his own misgivings, that he must convince his patients that one more medication trial is worth the effort, that one more stint at rehab will turn things around, that they will eventually attain some measure of relief. And finally, in his most artful sleight of hand, he must convince them that he himself believes in the healing process even as he questions his own prowess. But the doctor-protagonist depicted in these stories deserves the faith of his patients precisely because he refuses to be taken in by the authority and prestige of his profession. Of course, he realizes it would be cruel not to at least pretend. Thus, with maneuvers worthy of a shaman, he cajoles and encourages his patients to maintain their faith in the latest white powder while together they cling to the same lifeboat. Fittingly, in the title story, it is the patient who takes a turn at the helm and figures out that one need only add a methyl group to a useless old antihistamine and *voila*...the Spanish Molecule—the mythical balm that promises to restore the patient to health and provide the healer with a well-deserved respite. But even the Spanish Molecule, it turns out, carries a warning label. And so our doctor-narrator, this artful but embattled improviser, must again reckon with the limits of his dark arts. He must soldier on under the burdens of uncertainty. Both he and his unfortunate patients are the better for it.

−ROB GOLDSTEIN. MD

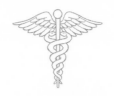

CASE ONE

WHY DO YOU LOOK AT HIM?

———————●———————

One of the greatest tricks parents play on children is to tell them that when they grow up, they can be whatever they want to be. Not only is this notion the height of foolishness, it is also exceedingly cruel.

*Rather than whip up this meringue, parents ought instead teach children, through example, how to avoid becoming **captive** to their choices.*

The problem is, most parents haven't themselves learned this lesson.

THE SETUP

Pamela Parker had a problem. For reasons not obvious to her, she recently developed a peculiar habit: slugging whiskey straight from the bottle. Several times a day. Every day. Secretly. Jameson.

I don't want to mislead. From Mrs. Parker's perspective, Jameson was not her actual problem. Were she honest with the world, Mrs. Parker would readily concede that her actual problem was *getting caught* slugging Jameson. In the middle of the day. During a holiday gathering with family. Two different gatherings, in fact.

And the family wanted her to stop. For every day thereafter.

This irked Mrs. Parker.

Robertson Parker had a problem. His wife, Pamela, could not stop slugging Jameson multiple times a day, every day, in secret. The reason behind this perplexed Mr. Parker; the behavior was *so* completely out of character. Had he lived in an earlier century, Mr. Parker might suspect a malignant *daemon* at play, such was the deviance of Mrs. Parker's actions from the woman he knew her to be. But supernatural causation was no longer in vogue in Mr. Parker's century, so he was left at a loss.

Interestingly, Mr. Parker's *first* response to the discovery of his wife's affection for Irish distillates was to, *de facto,* look the other way; he adopted a clamorous gait walking about their living quarters. Mrs. Parker therefore could hear him approach and deftly stash the Jameson, if it happened to be out at the time.

One could not entirely fault Mr. Parker his avoidance, tramping about heavy-footed like that, because he himself wasn't aware of his avoidance. A veil hung within his mind—a veil that cloaked his wife's relationship with Jameson. This happens sometimes when a person is confronted with something they don't want to see, even though they've plainly seen it. The brain figures a way to not see the already seen, like an accomplished sleight-of-hand artist. Of all the things Mr. Parker conjured up in his stream of consciousness, tellingly, the image of his wife with Jameson at her lips was nowhere to be found.

In his own way Mr. Parker operated like Mrs. Parker, who also put her Jameson fetish behind a veil—really more like behind a lead apron—to shield the bad business from her normal conscious deliberations. Left to their own devices, Mr. and Mrs. Parker might have lived this way happily ever after, amid yet not aware of the specter within their home. But there were other players who had a stake in the game, and they held significant leverage.

Dr. Hamilton Sinclair had a problem. He was on the phone with his longtime patient Robertson Parker and just learned that Mr. Parker's wife, Pamela—also his longtime patient—had recently resumed her clandestine habit of drinking room-temperature Irish whiskey directly from the bottle. And this was after her adult children had caught her at two family functions. Highly improper conduct. Dr. Sinclair, though invisible to Mr. Parker through the phone, raised his hand in a futile effort to interrupt. He had heard enough.

As Dr. Sinclair would shortly discern, Robertson Parker lived in a world where powerful men had special rules regarding language. For one thing, they never had to expressly ask for help. In Mr. Parker's case, he simply made statements and others knew what to do, which was usually something that he wanted done. After hearing the facts about Mrs. P.'s fixation with the bottle, Dr. Sinclair realized this was Mr. Parker's way of asking for help. Which is another way to say that he realized Mrs. Parker's problem was now his problem.

Dr. Sinclair had worked hard to create a genteel, upscale, professional medical office on Park Avenue near 84th Street in Manhattan. He counted wealthy families like the Parkers as his bread and butter, in part because they lived in the genteel and upscale neighborhood, but also because families like the Parkers were loyal to the professionals they engaged. Indeed, Dr. Sinclair knew that he enjoyed the same fealty as Mr. Parker's stockbroker—provided he generated similar returns on investment. This was one of those moments when Dr. Sinclair needed to deliver the goods.

Alcohol problems had not yet been eradicated from Park Avenue above 79th Street, but this was neither Dr. Sinclair's expertise nor his interest. Like many physicians attracted to medicine for the rewards it offered those who could reason clearly, he found addictive behaviors highly illogical, and not a small degree messy. Here was an excellent case in point. Dr. Sinclair could make no sense whatsoever of Mrs. Parker's drinking, and he had heard quite enough to glean the intra-family conflict it caused. With no insight to offer Mr. Parker as they spoke on the phone, the doctor admitted that Mrs. Parker's behavior made no sense to him either. It made no sense to anyone—and that's often when someone thinks of calling a psychiatrist.

———————•———————

I found myself with a new problem. Dr. Sinclair decided to outsource Mrs. Parker to fulfill his duty and passed the Jameson bottle to me. I was grateful for the gesture. Referrals like Mrs. Parker were my bread and butter, albeit for messy and illogical problems, but that was my choice after all. Sinclair had something on me though,

DANIEL MIERLAK, MD, PHD

something very important—he knew his patient. For me, she was another stranger knocking at the door.

Referrals from Dr. Sinclair promised a certain type of patient, that's true, but there's always an element of unpredictability in psychiatric work. The field recognizes this. For example, I'm pretty sure no other medical specialty explicitly suggests that when setting up an office, one ought to place the patient's seat closest to the door, just in case paranoid impulses urge a hasty exit. One wouldn't want to be between paranoia and the door. And why, if not for unpredictability's sake, do some psychiatrists' offices have a "panic button" that can signal an emergency to outside staff? Do cardiologists install this technology? To protect against that threatening heart murmur? Some patients themselves, after a consideration of the potential risks in my work, have suggested I keep a firearm in the office. Those patients always sit very close to the door.

Mrs. Parker would pose no threat to physical integrity, but that isn't the only risk in the job.

SESSION ONE

The forces of coercion must have been formidable because it was clear Pamela Parker didn't want to be having this conversation. There are various ways patients communicate when the arm is twisted. In Mrs. Parker's case, it was the quality of her response to my standard opening, "Now that we're together, tell me in detail what brings you in." Her recital, a combination of sentences and phrases, did not carry the smooth flow of ordinary narrative. It was more like a prepared statement for an allocution hearing.

"I'm drinking more than I should.

"I'm sixty-seven years old.

"I've been married forty-five years.

"I have four children.

"All Harvard or Yale alumni.

"Well-established now with their own families.

"My husband is a partner at Davis.

"We live on 89th Street.

"Also in Quogue.

"I suppose you'll want to know that my father died two years ago."

She was stiff, no one would disagree, but maybe that was a function of circumstance. I could see her dilemma. Mrs. Parker looked the part of a wealthy, Upper Eastside sophisticate. Her life script never included a scene at an addiction psychiatrist's office, copping to a problem with hitting the sauce too hard. The restraint she exhibited, with perfect posture, was expected from someone of her station. But, that tone? No one was born with that much vinegar in her. Nah, she was bullied into the visit—the delivery nailed it. I lurched forward with my second question.

"What do you mean 'drinking more than I should?'"

Mrs. Parker returned to the history. Her austerity relaxed an angstrom as she spoke extempore. For decades, she had the habit of pouring a small amount of whiskey into a liqueur glass before dinner. Infrequently, she would have some wine with the meal. The previous summer Mrs. Parker began a new pattern: she took a slug of whiskey directly from the bottle.

Gradually one slug led to another. Then, to daily slugs. Then, to frequent daily slugs. Then, to secret frequent daily slugs.

There was no explanation. Maybe loneliness since her father died, she speculated? Mrs. Parker provided doting care as he declined. The theory was plausible, even with the passage of a couple of years, but how about some emotional corroboration? Even a smidgen? I would never doubt sadness or loneliness after the loss of a parent, but man it was well hidden here. All I got from Mrs. Parker was the reflection of an outsized chip that sat there on her shoulder, and I knew enough to steer clear of that sucker. So maybe this was a good time for a third question?

"You were close?"

Mrs. Parker took some time on that one. She glazed over a bit and moved her head slightly left. That broke her line of sight off of me and planted it onto a nearby section of wall, a blank area of nondescript plaster. There she stared, lost in thought. I had been focused on her face all the while, but the pause allowed me to begin a serious study. After three decades of scrutiny, I have come to see that all faces have beauty within them, but not at all times. With the sheets of facial muscles tensed just so, Mrs. Parker projected anger, which wasn't a good look for her. I meandered around the neighborhood—the nostrils, the cheekbones, the right earlobe—then swung back to the eyes. *Wait, what was that?* Some barely perceptible change. Something with the eyes. *Oh, yes, I see it now.* Her lacrimal glands had hiked their fluid production. She was welling up.

"He was my biggest fan."

A few blinks and she mopped the spill. Whatever memory my question inspired was quickly dispatched back to storage. The moment had passed, and with it the softening that tears can produce. This appeared to be another topic Mrs. Parker wasn't eager to discuss. My gaze drifted down to her jaw line, which had regained its strength. She resumed her history.

Raised in affluence, Mrs. Parker did quite well in school, she wanted me to know. Robertson Parker's family had membership at her club. After they married, a pregnancy promptly followed, and she set aside her dream of graduate school to raise the children. It was a smart compromise; her husband stood out in law school, and then in the firm. Several decades later, Mrs. Parker could be found ensconced in the rarefied world of New York society, matriarch to a brood of overachievers and their aspiring progeny. There was nothing wrong with this picture. Well, almost nothing.

Enigmatic or not, secret drinking runs the risk of eventual discovery. For Mrs. Parker, it was an Easter luncheon that did her in. Her son-in-law observed the swig through a door left ajar. He didn't say anything that first time, undoubtedly confused by the juxtaposition of Jameson with Coco Chanel and Mikimoto. He was now on alert though, and after a second observation some weeks later he came forward—after all, there were grandchildren to think of. That conversation must have mortified Mrs. Parker. Even unspoken, as I'm sure it was, the implication that she might not be fit to watch her grandchildren…Scandalous.

Of course the indiscretion with whiskey would stop immediately.

A month or two later, she was back at it. Mr. Parker found an empty bottle and knew that, with his kids on the scent, the jig would be up soon enough. He called Dr. Sinclair, who heard the tale and punted to me.

Why *had* she resumed Jameson with so much now at stake? It was a damned good question. Alas, Mrs. Parker really had no idea. I was cool with that. We didn't need to know the "why" to make progress, we could just focus on the "what"—what to do about the unorthodox business.

I could tell Mrs. Parker didn't like her role in the doctor-patient dyad; she flashed that chip like this consultation was *my* fault. Nevertheless, she couldn't deny it was in her interest to figure out how to extricate Jameson from her life. I decided my next move should be to lay out the options for her quandary.

I launched into a review of the treatment options for problematic drinking of spirits, running the list like a waiter recites the specials. Mrs. Parker had no appetite for standard fare like group or AA. So instead, I improvised an off-menu, office-based treatment platter. It included behavioral ingredients (the removal of Jameson from the homes, the agreement to three months of abstinence), biological side dishes (medications for alcohol disorders), and finished in a psychological citrus-soy (efforts in therapy to identify triggers, explore life stressors, etc.). After the kitchen could offer no more, Mrs. Parker considered my "special" special.

"Well, the whiskey's already been removed from Long Island."

"Very good. The recommendation is to remove it from Manhattan in addition."

To that she demurred.

"Perhaps it could be moved to a hard to reach area."

Ahh...she wanted to leave the back door open a crack—not a good sign, but then I remembered waiters were not paid to negotiate. We continued to haggle over her order nonetheless. Mrs. Parker preferred to avoid medication options, but surprisingly did agree to three months of abstinence. As regards therapy, she was silent. It looked to be a pretty modest dish in the end—no Jameson in Quogue and an agreement to not drink for three months—but Mrs. P. was the customer, and that's all she had a hankering for.

Addiction treatment always has a starting point: the elements of the initial treatment plan. Mrs. Parker's initial plan was as tight as cheesecloth. More important than where one starts, though, is whether one has the willingness to adjust the plan based on results. I didn't have the stomach to raise the notion of an *upward* adjustment should she resume her tryst with Jameson. What I really could use was an ally—someone to act as a second set of eyes, a partner to help tag-team her when the empty bottles showed up in the trash.

"Might Mr. Parker want to join us to discuss the options?"

"I'm sure he would."

Lovely.

THE CLOSE

They returned together a few weeks later. Mr. Parker, a slim, distinguished-looking gentleman, was considerably less fretful than his wife. His presence did not have a calming effect, however. If anything, Mrs. Parker seemed wound tighter, were that even possible.

Mr. Parker chose to sit on the large chair rather than beside his wife on the loveseat. They had not discussed an agenda and looked to me for guidance. I thought we could start with Mr. Parker's view of the issue. He related the events of the past year at length. I commented that his account was in complete agreement with that of his wife.

Just then, somewhere deep inside Mrs. Parker, a river of magma moved a few inches.

"Well, I should hope so," she muttered sotto voce.

Wait, who was she talking to? Was that zinger meant for me? Apparently, the few weeks off softened nothing.

Mrs. Parker looked good and pissed, and itching for a fight, but with whom…And for what? With me, for the gall to vet her story? Or her husband, who threw her under the bus with Sinclair? Or the children, who really should just mind their own business? I could take my pick of the lot, but the last thing I wanted was to get into a catfight with her. I had no skin in this game. Also, I would lose.

Ten seconds went by with these cogitations—very long, silent seconds. I looked at Mrs. P., still as a stone, lips pursed as if to conceal a quarter-lemon. Then to Mr. P., unfazed.

It's the easiest thing to avoid a fight sometimes. Mr. Parker was expert and offered a model: just pretend not to notice.

"So…Mrs. Parker…How have things been going?"

That put us back onto agreeable ground. Mrs. P. had three discrete glasses of wine since our initial meeting, spread out across three different meals. That was her nonproblematic drinking. Mr. Parker interrupted and volunteered that for many years they drank together this way. He did not look at his wife as he spoke. They both clearly wanted to preserve this pattern. Mr. Parker said as much, but added, "as long as it doesn't risk the other drinking." I tried to explain how difficult it was to predict whether Mrs. Parker could drink wine moderately without eventual reversion to whiskey.

"So what are the options?" he asked.

Here was the opening I needed to establish control of the session. His question would allow me to don my professorial robe and issue forth on treatment options. But there was strategy to consider as well. If I played my cards right, Mr. Parker could become a useful confederate.

We would start with the exceedingly rational stratagem of removing alcohol from *both* homes, something Mrs. Parker only partially agreed to. I had to avoid direct confrontation with her resistance; feathers would ruffle for certain. It would be much better to have *Mr. Parker* realize, and say out loud, that *any chance* of access to Jameson in the Manhattan apartment spelled trouble. In this way we would function as a team: I set him up, and he delivers the punch line. It would then be two on one, and that might earn a concession from the unflappable Mrs. P. Some might wonder whether I was attempting a rather direct manipulation of the couple. Yeah, so? Manipulation isn't always a dirty word.

I looked at Mrs. Parker and remarked, "At the first visit, you mentioned Jameson had been removed from the house on Long Island. That's correct, right?"

Without waiting for her response I turned and looked directly at Mr. Parker, but before he could say anything, Mrs. Parker blew the magma.

"Why do you look at him?!"

Her tone, a scold, dazed me like a sucker punch. Then, she followed with a straight jab to the face.

"Why do you ask **me** and then look to **him** to answer??"

Shit. I'm here playing chess in my head and I blow the first move. It wasn't even the first move—I was just prepping the board. I simply wanted to corroborate that Jameson had been removed from Quogue as a setup for the Manhattan play. Instead, I implied Mrs. Parker *might be a liar*, and she wasn't taking to that kindly. I inadvertently dinged her bloody chip. A vigorous spray of adrenaline and cortisol shot out from my adrenal glands. Fight, flight, fear, shame—you name it—it was all there as the hormones surged. Machiavelli was laughing in his grave.

To finish, she cleaned my clock.

"I think if I said **I removed it**, that should be the end of it!"

There's just no way to tiptoe around this reality: it's nearly impossible to maintain decorum in a discussion about sneaking hard liquor.

It was time to enter damage control mode, once again, with yet another patient. Somehow, the spike of stress hormones did not completely overwhelm my cognitive faculties. That was good; I needed all the help I could get. As for my confederate Mr. Parker, he sat silent. Some ally.

I adopted an educational tone: "I apologize. Let me clarify. *The disorder* can induce deception, and so verification of facts is necessary. This says nothing of trustworthiness in general, which is not in question. It's just around behavior with Jameson—I wanted to corroborate the removal from Quogue. I understand this is difficult—no one likes to feel they aren't being trusted."

Mr. Parker sat poker-faced, but seemed to understand.

Mrs. Parker just sat poker-faced.

Mercifully, Mr. P. did what powerful men often do in moments of shared awkwardness—he changed the subject.

"I want to make sure we're doing everything we can."

I looked at Mrs. Parker. She was gone. Whatever tiny shard of authority I might have called upon was lost. That's not to say Mrs. Parker was about to storm out of the office offended, as other patients did at times. That wasn't her style by a long shot. She preferred to say nothing; the chip did all the talking. But it was clear she made up her mind to be done with me. She had the same look we all get towards salesmen who pitch unwanted services.

Fortunately, the session was nearly up. It had unraveled to a fairly comprehensive shambles, and that reminded me of those figure skaters in the Olympics who fall repeatedly in their final routine. Certain of failure, they soldier on nevertheless and finish their program. That's the spirit I needed to emulate. Mr. Parker had asked a question and, damn it, I would finish my answer. Discussion of the behavioral treatment lay in ruins, but there was still the therapy portion of the skate to complete.

Game face reassumed, I spoke of how events in one's life, or a stage of life, could cause emotional upheavals. Sometimes these emotions weren't easily accessible, but they were powerful and could contribute to behaviors like substance use. Conversations to explore whether Mrs. Parker's drinking was related to issues in her life could be useful.

Thud.

Mr. Parker stared back blankly. Mrs. Parker, who'd been staring blankly onto her favorite section of plaster, continued the same. They did not respond. Ouch. Then, just at that moment, as if to prove that everything is, in fact, absurd, I had the unhelpful thought arise that this would be a good time to stand and dance a little jig, like a jester might.

"I see the session is over," Mr. Parker finally declared, a fitting double entendre. "Thank you for your time, doctor."

He began to stand. Mrs. Parker and I followed suit. Handshakes and thanks were exchanged. It was strange, this ending, to be fired by a couple this way: one unspoken but blunt, the other cordial but indirect. I was unsettled by it all—my inability to develop a rapport, the sloppy blunder, and inept repair—and I felt compelled to say something, anything, as to not leave the last word ambiguous.

"So you'll let me know how you want to proceed."

Mrs. Parker had already exited the office but was still within earshot in the vestibule. She did not break her stride. Mr. Parker, behind her, was just at the door, his back to me. He stopped at my statement, stiffened, turned his head, and spat over his shoulder.

"I'll be getting back to you on that."

POSTSCRIPT

I didn't wait by the phone. That was smart.

But I kept thinking of the Parkers, whether I could have played it differently with them and somehow persuaded Mrs. Parker to come in for regular sessions.

Here's what I imagined:

If Mrs. Parker came in weekly, we could have spoken about her life for a while and not even bothered with Jameson at all, just had her tell her story. If she came to see me as an interested listener, her resistance might have lessened over time, and I might have come to learn other things about her in the process. Perhaps even earn her trust.

If I asked the right questions, I imagined Pamela Parker would tell me there was a soundtrack that played in her mind. This soundtrack was the inner monologue of her thoughts. It never stopped, this monologue; it rolled on and on. When lost in thought, Pamela mentally talked to herself, which turned the monologue into a dialogue of sorts. These thoughts were a part of her, naturally. Whose thoughts could they possibly be if not hers?

I imagined Pamela would agree that this inner dialogue was the uncensored story of what she privately reflected on. Oh, there was plenty of random chatter in there at all hours—much of it involved commentary on recent interactions, and planning for the future. But if I gained her trust, I suspected Pamela would fess up that certain themes bounced around in her head in particular.

Considering that hefty chip she lugged around, I was convinced a big one was that Pamela felt underappreciated.

I thought Pamela would agree with my conjecture, if based only on the inordinate time she spent lost in thought about this very subject. This train of thought would inevitably lead her to a singular conclusion: she was smart and talented, and capable—but for various reasons she was held back from a full realization of her potential.

The arguments here had a few pillars, I postulated.

In the first place, she was born female in a male-dominated world. I presumed that after a while Pamela realized no amount of raw merit would overcome the societal bad luck to be born a woman.

In the second place, I reckoned Pamela saw any chance for career fulfillment dashed when she agreed to subordinate to her husband's career, so he could climb the firm's ladder. The submission cost her everything professionally—and effectively nailed that coffin shut for good.

In the third place, I supposed Pamela felt that the world itself seemed uninterested in what she had to offer, what she could accomplish. The men she knew, starting with her husband, were thoroughly self-absorbed. And the women... were oblivious beyond their domestic concerns.

I figured the whole thing added up to a shit deal, when it could have been so much more.

Pamela, I speculated, talked to herself this way quite often. It was understandable. There was nothing about her gender, her marriage, or her social circle that was likely to change. I presumed all these predicaments led Pamela to think the same conclusion I did: she was underappreciated.

Even if true, no one ever heard those thoughts. They played like a broken record in her head for *decades*, but no one knew they existed. Except Pamela. And she wasn't talking. That wasn't her style.

Now, insofar as the rest of the world was concerned, I had a strong intuition there existed a *different* storyline as to who Pamela was. It was simple. It was based on what the world saw, what was plainly visible. To the rest of the world, Pamela was simply angry. This I could personally attest to.

Of course, no one in her world uttered a word of this to Pamela. It would be improper, impolite, and indelicate. This I could personally attest to. So Pamela had no idea how the world saw her. And, anyway, she had her hands full dealing with underappreciation.

How ironic about Pamela and her world. They were clueless to each other's perspective. This happens more than you know among people and the world they live in, whether in my imagination or not.

I suspected things had recently changed; I suspected Pamela's inner dialogue shifted focus. It became preoccupied with her dead father. I envisioned that Pamela found herself immersed in images from childhood, and of that last year caring for him. How a specific memory was chosen from the vast pool available was anyone's guess. Sometimes an association set one off, like hearing a song on the radio. Many others were mysterious in origin, just as vivid but summoned up for God-knows-what rhyme or reason.

It didn't take a great imagination to infer Pamela missed her father terribly. I saw it in her eyes for a second before she shoved that pain down. What did she say to me that moment as if in a trance? *"He was my biggest fan."* What else could that mean but that a father saw the truth about his daughter? I got the feeling maybe he was the only one. Now his eyes had gone opaque. Where did that leave her?

Alone.

With her smarts and talents, and capabilities—alone.

Sad, sad, and further sad. That's where the *new* inner dialogue took Pamela, I imagined, should anyone have dared ask. No one did. It would be improper, impolite, and indelicate.

Anyway, as I already concluded, the world had made up its mind as to who Pamela was. She hadn't ever changed. As far as the world saw, Pamela was simply angry.

And why not? The only person who knew the truth about her was dead.

It had never been fair. And it isn't fair.

And, in my imagination, that's when a slug of Jameson would come to Pamela's mind.

———————•———————

Is any of this accurate? Who knows? Maybe Pamela drank because she was a drunk.

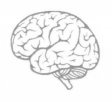

CASE TWO

THE LIMITS OF PERSUASION

———————•———————

In the old days, therapists and patients spoke of
agency*—the capacity to control the course of one's
life by self-reflection and reasoned action—as a
function that one could enhance with proper guidance and effort.*

*Nowadays, philosophers and scientists regard
agency as largely an illusion.*

ALTHOUGH I DIDN'T know it at the outset, by the time I started my work with Victor, the damage wrought to his life by anxiety and alcohol was beyond repair. Let me explain.

A full-blown hypochondriac, Victor often came to sessions and handed me a card, on which he had typed his name, the date, and a list of his current medications, with doses and directions—a *dramatis personae* of the pharmaceutical play staged within his body at that moment. If the point of typical hypochondria was to troll medical settings for reassurance over imagined illness, then Victor had a sadistic variant. He clearly did not imagine illness; Victor had numerous *actual* physical illnesses. Rather, Victor's hypochondriasis was concerned with worst-case scenarios. Which is to say it lent to the recurrent conviction that, as a result of what he was feeling, Victor had *fatal* illness.

Victor brought the typed card to appointments with other doctors as well, as a time-saving device. He preferred to spend the time with these doctors in argument that his symptoms, an assortment of mixed pathologica, meant he was dying, soon. And yet, for a guy this preoccupied with mortal disease, it was surely ironic that Victor hastened death by his own hand.

I refer to the liquor, of course.

———————•———————

Victor hadn't always been a hypochondriac, but since adolescence he had more or less always been an alcoholic. Don't cry for Victor, though—it wasn't a case of *all* bad genes. It never is. As if to balance his unwelcomed attributes, Victor was born with an exceptional intellect—a marvel that he freely exhibited. And one that attracted the attention of a certain kind of woman, like Missy, who eventually hitched her wagon onto Victor's and bore him four sons.

Alas, Victor took the gift of his intelligence for granted—a gift, I should point out, he had nothing to do with. Actually, it was worse than that. Beyond simple neglect to show gratitude for good fortune, Victor had the *chutzpah* to conclude it was his own decision to be brilliant, his own triumph. And worse still, in his calculus, those who didn't match his talents were of lower caste. It is true that Victor was smarter than most people he met, but why the zero-sum view of the world? Why, if he was the winner in the intelligence game, did everyone else have to be the loser?

Let's be clear and acknowledge that, in contrast to less accomplished narcissists, Victor's brilliance easily

DANIEL MIERLAK, MD, PHD

deduced the advantage to keeping one's superiority private. He never gave overt expression to his derision towards others. Thus astute, Victor dazzled in public performances and briskly climbed the corporate ladder. Born very smart, Victor learned how to become very successful, and began to accumulate wealth and prestige.

We should not focus on just these few traits when thinking of Victor. We really should add selfish to the list. How else can one understand his choice to drink *ad libitum* while Missy did all the heavy lifting to rear their four rambunctious boys? It was shameful. Don't get too angry with Victor, though—fate would again intervene to level out imbalance.

I refer to the liquor, of course.

———————•———————

I "got" Victor as a result of returning a call to a colleague who worked on the inpatient psychiatry unit at a top Manhattan hospital, where Victor had checked himself in seven days prior. The call was placed as the unit neared the end of its work, which for Victor meant a clean-out of his addictive drugs and replacement with nonaddictive drugs. Victor was slowly killing himself with alcohol so the concept made complete sense. But too often these days the *sole* focus of the psychiatric hospital is to simply change meds. Inpatient stays have become very short, too short to delve into puzzling aspects of a patient's life, like why, if they were so convinced of terminal illness, did they drink to the point of needing medical detox?

Don't get me wrong, playing with the chemical milieu of the brain can have profound positive effects. I just speculate whether other factors can be important for recovery. For example, I sometimes wonder how much the psychiatric hospital's power to heal comes from just removing the patient from their stressful environment. That's always explained a big chunk of why vacations work for me.

In any case, the unit was near the end of its work with Victor, and that meant someone needed to find outpatient resources for him, hence the call. I was an old hand at this drill, and I knew that multiple addiction psychiatrists would be called on Victor's behalf. My best chance to secure his entry into my practice was to respond quickly, as this transaction was often a first-come, first-served phenomenon. I looked at my calendar for the next week, saw it had some unwanted gaps, and called back with alacrity.

Lucky for me, my colleague answered his phone. Unlike the gravity of a psychiatric hospital admission, as seen from the perspective of the patient and family, the clinical handoff from hospital to outpatient psychiatrist could shock in its tepid superficiality.

"Oh yeah, hey, Dan, thanks for calling. We've got a guy discharging Friday, admitted about a week ago for extreme anxiety about his health. He's actually fine. He was self-medicating with alcohol and Klonopin. We detoxed him, tuned up his Lexapro and gabapentin, and he's ready to go. We're sending him to the Freedom Institute as well."

"Sounds good, I could see him Monday."

"Cool, what time?"

"I could swing 11 a.m."

"Excellent. I'll fax you the summary. Have a good weekend."

"Thanks, you too."

Forgive us our matter-of-factness. Repetition can make almost anything routine. Fear not, though; I would get my payback for being so ho-hum. Discharged Friday, Victor showed up at the office Monday 11 a.m. on the dot—hungover, tremulous, and convinced he was about to die.

———————•———————

It's hard to convey the challenge of sitting with Victor that first session. The normal conventions of my work— to obtain the history of the current complaint, the past history, the family history, the medical history—were upended by the man in the other chair. Waves of tears and great full-body shudders roiled his effort to speak complete sentences. He rarely made eye contact, but when he did I was taken aback by his stunning blue eyes, and by the desperation they called out. How does one clinically manage a stranger's desperation? I don't remember a class on that; I might've been sick that day.

Victor's misery demanded attention, as much as a crushed limb demands morphine. Nothing mattered but relief of pain. This dynamic would pervade many sessions to come—together we would lock onto the ultra-present, namely the inner torment experienced by Victor that very second. I could hear him stammer, but more arresting was to see him suffer just a few feet away. The scene rendered an inquiry into specifics difficult—in the same way that it is difficult to find out exactly how a limb got crushed when the patient is screaming in pain. Difficult, but not impossible.

I forced Victor to focus on my questions, cutting him off repeatedly until he gave a satisfactory answer, and I ignored for the moment his emotional pyrotechnics. It must have seemed cold from a psychiatrist, my disregard for his psychic pain, but I needed clinical data to help him lest I get sucked into his stupefaction. The tactic worked, Victor submitted to my interrogation, and its effect was to distract him away from raw panic and towards the information I sought. Gradually, he calmed enough to provide some history.

Victor relapsed to copious vodka over the weekend, less than twenty-four hours after discharge from the hospital that shored him up. Other facts spilled forth: he was rudderless after a breakup, reeling in unemployment, strung out over a son on heroin, and convinced his heart was about to blow. Victor's need to quell his exquisite anxiety was relentless, and it made forays into these topics brief and unsatisfying. Nevertheless, I was able to stitch together this proto-narrative:

Victor was single. Missy, grown fatigued of her status as a virtual single mom, dumped him over the drinking years ago and became a factual single mom. After that, Victor embarked on a series of highly dependent relationships with women. The last one ended a few months ago and contributed to Victor's current crisis.

Victor had ascended to apex executive levels within his industry, this despite the habit of consuming large volumes of vodka at all hours. Eventually confronted for "alcohol on breath" by his CEO, the only man above him in the org chart, Victor inexplicably resigned rather than take a leave of absence for a plush rehab. His plan to call some contacts and pivot into a highly paid consultancy, exempt from HR policies on substance use, was smashed to bits against the storm surge of his encroaching anxiety.

Victor was estranged from all his sons except Ned, a professional heroin addict whose lifestyle lit up Victor's fears like a Christmas tree. All these circumstances, combined with Victor's own maladies—diseases of the heart, blood, and GI tract—produced a pile of super-dry kindling ready for a spark.

In short, Victor was a hot mess.

Like many patients I've worked with, Victor's intellect was a force of nature and far surpassed my own. In and of itself, however, a five-star brain isn't necessarily enough to keep one out of all forms of trouble. Even the most brilliant man cannot think himself out of severe mental illness or addiction, although he can certainly think himself *into* terrible decisions just as frequently as the rest of us. That's why a high IQ ain't everything. Victor had his hands in plenty of trouble. I didn't need to win a pissing contest over IQ to treat him, I just needed the wit to persuade him to make choices for the better, or at least based in reality.

Easier said than done.

LIMIT NO.1: WHEN THE VOICE OF REASON FALLS ON DEAF EARS.

Between his spirited anxiety at baseline and vodka's enhancement, Victor had enough adrenaline dissolved in his blood to convince him of an imminent cardiac catastrophe. But fortunately reason had not escaped my office entirely, and it reminded me there *was* the little fact that the guy had just gotten released from a week's admission at a premier Manhattan teaching hospital.

"Victor, did you have a medical workup at the hospital?"

"Yes," he quivered.

"Was it negative?"

"Yes," he sputtered, quivering.

"Then you're not about to die."

I would have this kind of brief, Socratic exchange with Victor on many occasions, and with regard to a variety of symptoms. My effort had little effect. Something happened to Victor when he felt ill in a certain way. He lost the ability to use rational operations to evaluate his feeling-state—a state that told him he was to die shortly. One can imagine how disconcerting that must have been. I'm sure in the moment it could easily disable the operations of rational thought. What made no sense though was that, try as I might to reassure him, Victor could never come to learn that he repeatedly misinterpreted the seriousness of his body's signals. They would trick him every time. Doubting his doctors' cool logic, he would leave their offices unpersuaded, then return home and ruminate on how much time he had left.

In that initial meeting I didn't yet know the depth of Victor's hypochondria, so I took the hospital's word on his medical integrity and pushed forward. It seemed to me that the first order of business as his newly sworn psychiatrist was to dial Victor's anxiety gauges out of the red zone. I said as much to conclude the session, predicting with confidence (and a healthy dose of suggestion) that we could achieve this together. As for the other complexities in Victor's life, I bypassed comment. They would require longer discussion. I gave Victor new medication instructions and sent him home.

LIMIT NO. 2: ARGUING AGAINST A DISTINCTION THAT MAKES NO DIFFERENCE.

Among the recommendations Victor received from me at the end of the first visit was to stop vodka. This suggestion seemed self-evident. We discussed various strategies to achieve this goal, including his referral to the Freedom Institute, an outpatient drug and alcohol center in Manhattan. Victor was no rookie to this process—doctors and counselors had given similar dictates before. However, Victor surprised me in the second session when he revealed that, after the consultation, he switched to drinking wine in the evening. I wouldn't have wagered on that; in my experience the more desperate the patient in alcohol withdrawal, the more likely he is to follow my instructions, at least initially.

Victor also announced he had no intention of following up with Freedom Institute. He said it simply wasn't necessary, wine never got him into trouble before, and he was delighted to report it served to take the edge off quite nicely. Vodka, he agreed, had to be avoided, but he felt pretty good the last few nights after a couple glasses of rosé with dinner, and he figured he would just cruise at that altitude.

Victor did look much improved and felt a whole lot better compared to our last meeting. How much my medication changes played a role was hard to say, but it was impossible not to notice that Victor had undergone a metamorphosis. He transformed from a vibrating blob of fear into a bold, confident speaker. Whatever the cause, the interval between sessions did him well—Victor was firmly back in the saddle, ready to follow his logic regarding wine. I envied his certainty; however, in this case, his belief as to the benignity of rosé was difficult to support. I could easily think of clinical, historical, statistical, and culinary objections. The hypothesis begged peer review.

"Uh, Victor, you just got out of the hospital for an alcohol-fueled, health freak-out over something that turned out to be nothing. You sure rosé is a good idea? Alcohol has a way of getting ahead of itself. I think you've seen that."

"Never with rosé. It is a delicate flower compared to the cudgel of Grey Goose. I sip it before my appetizer. Think of it as a *digestif*."

"How about we think of it as ethyl alcohol—you know, the simple combination of carbon, hydrogen, and oxygen that landed you in the ER."

"That was the vodka, my friend, and that was my mistake. I shan't make the error again."

To that, Victor watched one of my eyebrows start to rise. He did not mistake the meaning, and he was not pleased. In response, he flashed his baby blues, now fiery, and betraying no shred of desperation. One might presume Victor knew perfectly well those cerulean eyes of his could be used to gin up an air of command, and in this case one would be correct. I wasn't, however, in a mood to submit, so I stared right back at him with my own Slavic green blinkers, and we faced off silently: tick, tick, tick. Victor flinched first, but ultimately showed who had the upper hand.

"I'll tell you what, if I falter with rosé I'll ring up your comrades at Freedom."

LIMIT NO.3: THE INABILITY TO ISSUE A MONEY-BACK GUARANTEE.

I would bide my time with Victor and his rosé. Time would ultimately judge whether his consumption remained a hobby or careened into compulsion. Meanwhile, our attention turned to the relationship with Ned, a topic Victor foamed to discuss. This dialogue, I must confess, felt distinctly like entering a theater an hour and a half late. The disorientation was brief, however, since it quickly became clear Victor's narrative was circular, in the sense that the action he described cycled around a repeating loop. One could enter the conversation anywhere and eventually be carried through every scene back to the point where one started. Ned was a career heroin addict who lived by his wits on the street—until he called Victor for help, and that's as good a place as any to begin the sequence.

It went something like this:

Ned would call in extremis pleading for a place to crash, and Victor would beg him to go to detox. Ned refused, and then moaned how depressed and suicidal he was. Victor could not handle that. He'd cut Ned off and tell him to come over, feebly insisting there would be conditions this time, like how long he could stay, that he couldn't steal, etc. Ned didn't have to be asked twice. He gorged on Victor's generosity for a while, violated all the conditions, and then disappeared with cash, checks, or easily sold objects under his arm. Time passed, Victor's burns healed, and Ned would call again. The wheel takes another turn.

"Victor, you realize you're facilitating Ned's addiction."

"And what would you suggest I do when he won't go into treatment?"

"He might not go into treatment because he knows you'll cave. What do you think will happen if you stand firm and refuse to let him come over?"

Victor started to look sick. He slipped into that lip-quiver I saw in the first visit. What followed came out shaky and rote, a dead giveaway he'd considered my question many times before.

"I've tried that…He starts talking about the depression…How bad it is…He's got nothing to live for…He's going to do it…He's going to overdose and end the pain..." Victor paused and time stopped for a bit.

"I can't have that."

I assumed Victor loved his son and shuddered at the thought of losing him. I'll always give the benefit of the doubt on that. But Victor's death anxiety by proxy was caught up with another issue as well: the problem of responsibility. As we spoke it became clear Victor could not tolerate the thought of complicity in Ned's death. The guilt he would experience if Ned died on the street, after his rebuff, set the anxiety turbines awhirl. And this is not to mention the implicit guilt for having shot tainted, addiction-prone DNA in his contribution to Ned's genesis. It all served to bring

Victor to the same terrible dread—a dread that had to be quashed by whatever means available. In this case alcohol wouldn't suffice, but opening his apartment door would.

So many times I've wondered how the tough-love pundits hedge this risk, that to withhold engagement could put the addict in greater harm's way. Families often worry whether cutting off their addicted loved one will lead to jail or death. While the former is an unpleasant but possibly transformative experience, the latter outcome leaves little to play with. How could I assure Victor he didn't have to worry about Ned dying in the street if he didn't open his door?

I couldn't.

Fortunately, there is a clinical bail-out strategy one can resort to when confronted with a complex, multifaceted, seemingly insolvable problem: find some part which *can* be addressed and organize around that. I latched onto the need to get Ned off the street, and I knew of a treatment center upstate that catered to difficult cases. As we both began to brainstorm how Ned might be cajoled towards this facility, Victor perked up with enthusiasm. But from what he described, my recommendation would be a temporary rest stop at best. Ned had many treatment episodes under his belt—episodes that ended prematurely because of disagreements with the treatment team. In addition to the proclivity for addiction, it was a good bet Ned also inherited his father's intellectual talents, and stubbornness.

LIMIT NO.4: WHEN THEY JUST DON'T WANT TO GO THERE.

Having hatched the plot to contain Ned upstate, we shifted to another of Victor's domestic concerns, namely the recent failed relationship with Cynthia, his former girlfriend. Cynthia fled for calmer waters after Victor impulsively resigned his job and began the anxious descent that would invigorate his drinking. The move away from Victor's recklessness was a sure sign of Cynthia's mental stability, but for Victor it meant losing hold of that rope that runs alongside a life raft. As he flailed, Victor's attempts to grab onto Cynthia became pure harassment, and she responded with a call to the police and issuance of an order of protection.

There were few levers to pull here with regard to options. To keep away from his ex-girlfriend made the only clinical, and legal, sense. That left us with the task of examining Victor's obsession with Cynthia, a mental process that isn't easily suppressed, even in the face of a court order.

"Victor, I imagine Cynthia became frightened by your relentless texts begging her to meet you and move back in."

"She overreacted. Had she given me a chance to explain my plan for consulting, she needn't have worried for the future."

"That a judge agreed with her suggests she wasn't overreacting."

"What can I tell you, doctor? The world has gone mad."

"I'm concerned you'll have impulses to contact her again. That's the way this thing goes. You can't just clear her from memory. We should make a plan for what to do when the urges come back. There's a lot at stake for you."

"Thank you for your vote of confidence. I'm not an idiot. I won't do anything stupid."

And with that, Victor closed the door on any further discussion of Cynthia, and we raced off to the next anxiety.

LIMITS NOS. 5, 6, AND 7: ET CETERA, ET CETERA, ET CETERA.

I could write about Victor's difficulty moving to a smaller apartment in an effort to downsize (hint: he couldn't get it together to pack). Or his need to drop consulting and find a corporate job to earn money (hint: he couldn't get it together to interview). Or how, in short order, his anxiety mushroomed and flipped the hypochondria switches on again (hint: his heartburn heralded death within three months). It may be an overstatement to compare this to battle with the multiheaded Hydra, but at the least I sure felt like I was playing whack-a-mole.

LIMIT NO. 8: WHEN YOU REALIZE YOU NEVER HAD A CHANCE.

It dawned on me that, if the goal was to feel better, I was working towards it *way* harder than Victor. For all the lament about anxiety, Victor mustered little movement when presented with concrete action items. I took on each of his predicaments, made suggestions, and then received various noncommitments in exchange. How to understand this? Was Victor following his own genius master plan? Was he too raked with anxiety to act? Or lazy at heart? Did he just want to drink? It was pointless to ask any of these questions. Victor could answer them no more insightfully than a cat could remark on its motives to play with string.

Did it matter what label one tagged Victor with? Call him self-defeating, or anxious, an alcoholic, or narcissistic—the reality was that Victor was all these things and more. And yet even at the worst moments, even when the burden of Victor's infirmity reduced him to a jiggling bowl of Jello, somewhere inside one element never wavered. It was the conviction that, as a result of intellectual superiority, Victor always knew better—and its corollary, that he should therefore always follow whatever his intuition concocted.

At the end of the day, that's what mattered most for my purpose—Victor did what Victor wanted to do, regardless the counsel or the consequence. He continued to drink, even though I made a damn good case alcohol boosted his anxiety, which boosted his heart rate, which he interpreted as cardiac collapse. He continued to obsess over Cynthia, then ignored common sense and staked out her apartment at night, hoping to catch a glimpse—*and then what? What possible good would come from that?*

This treatment, I could argue, was a futile exercise. Not that it didn't have a purpose—treatment always has a purpose, even if bewildering to the doctor. It's just that in this case the futility made any purpose hardly worth the effort. The truth was, the treatment had become yet another repeating saga in Victor's life, with me in tow. Round and round and round we went, visiting the stations of anxiety in sequence, impotent to induce any change. It didn't matter the session, because eventually all the anxieties would come 'round again. This ride wasn't fun anymore; indeed it never was. The question was whether and how it might end.

———————•———————

What became of Ned, one might ask right about now? Ned dropped off the radar after admitting into the program upstate, a welcomed relief given the other anxieties in play. True to form though, Ned got himself kicked out of the one-year program at the two-month mark, for oppositionalism. He tooled around New England for a while, exploiting his charm to exact charity from various impressionable young ladies. In the back of my mind, I knew that if (when) Ned called upon Victor again, when his charm ran dry or the women ran dull, Ned would fire up Victor's anxiety as sure as a boiler whose pilot still burns. Rather than prepare for that possibility, which would have been prudent, I chose instead to cross that bridge when I came to it, which is a metaphorical way to say I preferred to avoid the whole thing altogether.

The party started to end in earnest when Ned made his predicable call to Victor. He was already on a bus back to the city, money gone, a line of teary women in his wake. Ned would need a shower, laundry, some meals, a bed, and a haircut, to begin with. I felt sorry for Victor when that call came in. He held so much hope that the program could turn Ned around. But that hope was dashed by Ned's inability to resist his impulses, regardless of their self-destructive consequences. *Hmm, where have I heard that story before?*

Victor didn't stand a chance. He couldn't risk Ned dying in the street, even if Ned chose that risk over and over, and he couldn't talk Ned into self-preservation. So he took him in again, and that wheel started its spin anew.

As bad as his circumstances were prior to Ned's return, after that bus pulled in from Holyoke, Victor proved the adage that things can always get worse. He sank to a new low and returned to vodka normally kept on lower shelves, consuming it around the clock. At that level of drinking one does not make plans or complete tasks, or attend to bodily care, beyond excretion and the need to vomit.

Victor was turning into an alcoholic version of Ned. The problem in the long run, and even in a long bender, is that alcohol is far more toxic than heroin. So, after weeks of matching Ned round for round, alcohol vs. heroin, Victor came to a perfect equipoise. This is the state, familiar to many AA attendees, when one becomes equally terrified of intoxication *and* withdrawal—when one can't imagine another drink *and* can't imagine stopping—simultaneously. It's just the kind of dilemma that can bring the most recalcitrant drinker to consider treatment, and that is precisely what happened. Victor checked himself into a clinic for medical detoxification.

I heard he took the deluxe package and stayed a month longer for inpatient rehab. I got that information second hand because, as far as I was concerned, after Ned came back, Victor vanished.

I would never see him again.

DANIEL MIERLAK, MD, PHD

POSTSCRIPT

Victor's departure allowed me to step out and see things from a bird's-eye view. I pictured Victor within the loops of anxiety his existence had become. Like great tornadoes they crisscrossed his landscape, plucking up those who got too close. Cynthia opted out of the maelstrom. I was eventually lost to attrition. Ned, for his own reasons, jumped *into* the vortex when his turn came. Yes, the picture had sharpened, but in the end my final image was of a tattered Victor, alone, sucked up into the monster funnel—doomed, and clinging on for dear life.

Long after my grim vision faded, I had the occasion to call my colleague Dr. G., a talented internist I've collaborated with for years. I sent Victor to him early on, after I realized the hypochondria required a team approach. We discussed another case, and when that was done I asked whether he had seen Victor recently.

"Oh, you haven't heard? I'm sorry. Victor died months ago. I hadn't seen him in some time. He stopped making appointments."

I was not shocked by the news, just curious. "How did you find out?"

Dr. G. had gotten the kind of inquiry every internist knows means a patient died.

"They called me from the eye bank."

Huh. I wouldn't have pegged Victor as an eye donor. He was so suspicious of his organs.

People can surprise you.

DANIEL MIERLAK, MD, PHD

CASE THREE

SUPERMODEL

———————•———————

Those who love an addict better have thick skins.

To be neglected in favor of a drug does a number on self-confidence.

ELENA TOLD ME that a bespectacled older man—a professional talent scout—initially spotted her out on the *rambla* of Montevideo. I've never been to Montevideo, or any part of Uruguay for that matter, so I could not picture Elena on that storied, oceanfront promenade. Instead, her statement triggered a memory: the time I bumped into a retired older man in Central Park—an amateur ornithologist—who told me he had just spotted a belted kingfisher in the Ramble. I have no doubt that for both men the chance rendezvous made their day.

Elena was fourteen when identified. That talent scout must have had a silver tongue, for he convinced Elena's parents she should travel to Japan to undergo training and begin a career. Raised by God-knows-who, an ocean away from her family, Elena proved the scout correct and blossomed into a stunning supermodel.

To sit with Elena now, nearly ten years since detection, was strangely ordinary—that is, until you looked at her. Taking all the features together, Elena's personage certainly elicited the readout "elemental beauty," but there was something else about the three-dimensionality of the experience with her that made it unique. It took a few sessions to figure it out, but I finally realized what made Elena different was that there was no angle of observation in which she wasn't flawless.

I came to see that Elena had a kind temperament. Surprisingly deferential, she had the habit of purposely extending her hand forward every time we stood at the end of appointments. I obliged the universal offering, and as we concluded she shook my hand a beat longer than necessary. Probably cultural I thought, but I took the courtesy to suggest a depth to her that could easily be overlooked among those beguiled by a one-dimensional perspective.

The problem was insomnia; her boyfriend stressed her out. He favored cocaine too much and made love to her not enough. This was mystifying, and made me suspicious I might have seriously underestimated the corrosive properties of cocaine all this time. I found some medicine that helped Elena sleep.

Later, as her twenty-fourth birthday approached, Elena became sad. She explained that after twenty-four, models fell out of the elite class and could no longer command the high-end jobs—jobs that paid ten thousand euro a day. She wasn't crying about the reduction in her day rate.

Once, Elena mentioned off-handedly that she was on the cover of the current issue of a fashion mag I had never heard of. As it happened, that night I was to meet some friends for dinner in the East Village. I arrived early, and while sauntering to the restaurant I passed a hipster shop common below 14th Street—just the kind of shop that carried obscure, elitist, specialty periodicals. I went in and found her issue.

The cover, Hubble-like in resolution, showed Elena in tight close-up: perfect hair, perfect skin, perfect makeup, perfect lighting, perfect features.

It didn't begin to do her justice.

POSTSCRIPT

Elena dropped out of treatment abruptly. She got a bunch of back-to-back bookings in Europe at a very high per diem, effectively causing her to move there for the immediate future. Which she did, after she dumped her boyfriend.

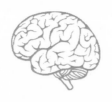

COIN OPERATED

For those who partake, not every altered state of consciousness is due to the drug.

On its very own the brain is more than capable of taking us on a long, strange trip.

HAROLD STOOD NAKED in the bathroom in a kind of torpor, waiting for the shower to get good and hot, knife at his side. It was a paring knife, selected from the appropriate drawer in the kitchen. The object optimized the properties Harold sought for his purpose: size, shape, and ease of cutting flesh.

This was not the first time Harold brought the knife into the bathroom and turned on the shower, intending to open a vein and exsanguinate while hot water rained down. Obviously, those prior efforts were aborted. An inhibition took hold and prevented the deed. Today felt different though—today the yen to be dead was irresistible.

Just twenty minutes earlier, while Harold was driving around town on errands, the urge came into existence. At first pure feeling, it spread like a hit of intravenous heroin and caused a warm shudder. The sensation lingered a minute, during which Harold seamlessly entered a dissociative trance and conjured a thought: get the knife and go to the shower. He obeyed.

Strange as it sounds, there *can* be a feeling, that leads to a thought, which leads to an intention, that leads to an action, whose outcome supposes self-annihilation. This sequence can proceed as if obligatory. And so it did.

———————•———————

Harold spent the better part of his sentience inhabiting an inner world devoid of basic, positive emotional states: pleasure, contentment, passion, and joy, to name a few. As sad as this was, a silver lining made all the difference—Harold was unaware of what he lacked, and so carried on ignorant of his fate. This all changed in high school, when Harold began to realize he operated differently from his peers.

It was a simple conclusion to draw. His friends did the same things Harold did—they were musicians, played varsity sports, and were excellent students. But when they spoke of these endeavors, Harold heard his friends convey enjoyment; they experienced positive feelings from the engagement. The contrast to Harold's un-experience couldn't have been clearer, and thus Harold began to see himself in a new light, a very unfavorable light—a defective, broken light.

Unwittingly depressed until then, Harold now became quite consciously depressed. He struggled on and off for years, and descended several times to that place that seeks nonexistence. He landed in my office a few days after the last foray to the shower. As often occurs, it was another pretext that prompted the consultation, something about a parent finding a bunch of empty beer bottles under his bed. But very quickly Harold dropped a dime on himself and came clean about how he ended up in the bathroom with the paring knife.

I could see he had no injury to his arms so I addressed the discrepancy directly.

"How come you're not dead?"

Harold answered, flatly, "We have this bench in the shower. I heard a noise…I heard something hit the bench…It sounded like a coin.

"I turned around and saw a penny on the bench."

"A penny? A penny fell onto the bench in the shower? Where did it come from?"

He kept a straight face, "It must have been stuck to my ass. Probably sat on it in the car somehow."

"A penny fell off your ass and landed on the bench." Saying it out loud only added to the wonder. "Why didn't you carry on with the knife?"

He paused between sentences, carefully reviewing the memories one by one. I could swear he got a little glassy-eyed.

"I didn't know where the penny came from at first…

"I stared at it awhile…

"I kind of came to…

"After that…" He blinked a few times and straightened up.

"I didn't feel like it anymore."

Strange as it sounds, there *can* be a feeling, that leads to a thought, which leads to an intention, that leads to an action, whose outcome supposes self-preservation.

POSTSCRIPT

I diagnosed Harold with chronic depression and suggested a trial of the antidepressant Wellbutrin. There was no resistance to the idea. Harold had an excellent response to the medicine and discovered who he was when not infirmed by clinical depression. There never was an alcohol problem.

He ended up leaving for Albuquerque, for a job in digital sales.

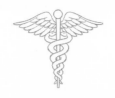

DOCTOR... I THINK I'M A MONSTER

———————◆———————

It's an old cliché, I know, but it's true—if you want to make it to the show, you've got to be able to hit the curve.

DOROTHY LIVED A rather uncomplicated life in Queens. She and her husband, Fred, shared traditional values and agreed, early in their marriage, that Fred would work while Dorothy raised the children. They had three daughters in all, spread out in a way that kept Dorothy busy for years. After her children grew up, Dorothy waited for them to produce their own children, and then helped to raise the next generation.

One of Dorothy's great joys was to spend time with her grandchildren. Her daughters lived nearby, which allowed for frequent babysitting and sleepovers. Dorothy discovered the secret sauce to a close relationship with adult kids who are parents—don't meddle in child-rearing practices.

Fred and Dorothy were avid smokers as young adults, as were many of their peers. Fred managed to quit with the arrival of children, but Dorothy would not follow suit. Over the years the family often encouraged her to quit, and now that young grandchildren were in the mix, her daughters became more insistent. Every time Dorothy came in from sneaking a smoke outside, they gave her the hairy eyeball.

Like many smokers who try to quit on their own, Dorothy repeatedly fell back into the addiction. The threat to her relationship with the grandkids demanded a different approach. After speaking with a friend who used a psychiatrist to quit cigarettes, Dorothy found her way to me.

I reviewed the strategies for smoking cessation. Dorothy was keen on the use of nicotine replacement; the logic made sense to her, and she liked the fact that the products were over-the-counter. She felt most comfortable to start with a simple regimen of nicotine patches along with some behavioral adjustments.

We met periodically to review her experience. Dorothy's smoking went from a steady pack-a-day to a sporadic pack-a-week. We examined the circumstances under which she gave into urges to light up and brainstormed countermeasures. Dorothy was a very motivated patient and did all her homework. She was pleased with her progress and saw complete abstinence within reach. Her daughters were also pleased, and the tension with them eased up greatly. Always the proud grandmother, Dorothy would not leave without telling me what her grandkids were up to, and what travel plans or art projects she had in the works for them.

Then, one time, in the middle of a session, Dorothy took pause and turned serious. She had said nothing to raise any red flags. I waited for her to speak.

"Doctor, I have to tell you
   something."

                              Tears began to well.

"Something is terribly
   wrong with me."

                              I sat upright.

"I haven't been able to
   tell anyone."

                         This was something big.

"I can't believe it."

                              Very big.

"I'm so scared."

                         She started to weep softly.

And not speak.

                         She stopped speaking.

I waited…

                              and waited…

and waited some more.

                              Until I could wait
                                 no longer.

"Dorothy?"

She wouldn't look at me.

"Dorothy, what is it?"

She opened her mouth.

"I…"

"I…"

The sentence would not form.

I sat still.

And waited.

Until it came.

Like birth following labor.

"I…"

"I…"

"I…"

"When I give the little ones a bath…"

She swallowed.

"I imagine I could drown them."

Tears unabated.

"Hold them under
 the water…"

The mouth twists sick.

"And watch them drown."

                              The physiognomy
                                  of revulsion.

"I love them so much…"

                              The physiognomy
                                   of shame.

"But this horrible scene…"

                              The physiognomy
                                 of loathing.

"I'm afraid what I might do."

                                      Her lip—

No, her whole face—

                                    Trembling.

"Doctor…"

                               Listen closely.

"I think I'm a monster."

*OK, that was enough; this had to be nipped in the bud
right now. I had been through this kind of thing before.*

"Dorothy, look at me."

                                  She did not.

"You're not a monster."

No movement.

"You don't want to hurt
your grandchildren."

Nothing.

"And you *won't* hurt your
grandchildren."

To that she looked up.

"You're having a classic
intrusive, obsessional
thought."

She wiped at an eye.

"These are unwanted
thoughts that pop into
our heads."

Then, the other eye.

"They're often of a violent nature."

The quivering stopped.

"Everybody has these
once in a while."

I paused.

Bewilderment befell.

"Other people have these thoughts?"

"I hear about them all the time. There are a million different examples. The first one I remember was before I became a psychiatrist, when I did research. A good friend who worked in a lab down the hall called me frantic. He was standing next to his boss when the thought occurred that he could pick up a nearby beaker and smash the boss's head. My friend was mortified.

"There are so many others. Someone watches a train pull into a station and thinks, 'I could jump on the tracks right now and be run over.' Or if the platform is crowded and a person in front is standing at the edge, the thought could appear, 'If I pushed her right now, she'd be killed by the train.' Or how about one that occurs to me once in a while? I'm driving on a highway and a tractor-trailer is approaching when I sometimes think, 'I could cut the wheel hard at the last second and plow right into the guy.'

"Think of it this way. There's deliberate thought, like when we sit down to plan an activity or a trip. But there are also random thoughts that just pop into our head unconnected to any train of deliberate thought. It's as though our minds have a thought generator that we're not aware of, that spits out weird stuff occasionally, often with very violent themes."

Dorothy stopped crying.

"I won't act on them?"

"They have nothing to do with how you feel about your grandkids, and they have no power over your actions. Just imagining these scenes will not make you act them out. They are fleeting thoughts thrown out by the generator.

"Believe it or not, these kinds of thoughts are completely normal experiences. Disturbing, yes. Unwanted… of course. Repetitive…quite often. All of this freaks people out. You can be sure your friends aren't bringing up their own examples in conversation."

We talked some more, and eventually Dorothy regained her composure. I sent her back into the world less afraid of her thoughts, I hoped—especially the ones she couldn't control.

Dorothy came back a few months later for her scheduled follow-up visit. She was excited. The intrusive images of drowning had stopped—vanished without a trace! Bath time was no longer filled with dread, just giggles and splashes. Overjoyed, Dorothy had become freed from her mental torment. She still hadn't spoken to anyone about this, even her husband, so I was the only person she could celebrate with.

"Doctor, I think it's a miracle."

POSTSCRIPT

Even I hadn't foreseen such a dramatic response for Dorothy—usually these kinds of intrusions persist to some extent. After understanding the nature of the "generator," however, one can flick those thoughts away like a pesky gnat. Dorothy was very lucky to have completely lost the drowning imagery given how often she had those grandkids in the tub. Whatever the reason for her good fortune, I happily took her response as a win.

She had those intrusions dead in the water.

THE SPANISH MOLECULE

How shall we judge a man—by what he is, or by what he does?

I'm told that great statesmen, for all the good they do to steer humanity from disaster, are often terrible fathers.

And we know mothers love their sons, even those who commit murder.

ALL THINGS CONSIDERED. Lindhoff might have preferred being born without a bent for the mechanical.
But, like all of us, he had no choice in the matter: one
does not *decide* one's preferences—one *discovers* one's
preferences. And for Lindhoff, there was no question
it just felt good to tinker, to take apart and put back
together, to learn from assembly, to make operational,
to create objects, and to experience function. What
could go wrong with such a practical predisposition?[1]

His passion was plain as day. As a preteen, Lindhoff
hunched over a workbench for hours on end, fiddling
with the latest kit for a remote-controlled something
or other—car, truck, boat, whatever. The activity put
Lindhoff into that special state of flow that comes with
the enhanced focus of singular effort: time stops, and all
else falls away. The flow state is reinforcing, not because
it produces a temporary euphoria, but rather because
it suppresses a chronic anxiety—the endless 'woulda,

---

1   Anything can go wrong under the right circumstance.

coulda, shoulda' of the mind's inner monologue. Deep levels of directed attention could, during flow, turn off self-conscious chatter in the head, and that's what *really* felt good.

Lindhoff did not see this at the time—he was just a kid who liked the feel of a soldering gun in his hand. As he grew older, the need and the satisfaction grew as well, from simple kits to complex machines: appliances, electronics, engines. Always creations he could hold and see in action.[2]

When it came time for Lindhoff to plan for college, he poked around and learned some schools offered engineering degrees, which is to say they taught students how to solve complicated problems. This appealed to Lindhoff for obvious reasons. Much of his free time was already spent assembling and dissembling machines others had invented to solve complicated problems. Couldn't he make a profession of it?

There were issues to consider here, however. Lindhoff clearly had a head for how parts formed the whole, but he had problems at school. He was not a good student in the classroom, at least as defined by later twentieth-century educators, who favored models of learning over learning from models. None of this ever caused Lindhoff noticeable grief though; there wasn't much he cared less about

---

2   When Lindhoff described his crowning achievement as the construction of a 3-D printer from scratch, it wasn't because of the complexity of the build. It was because he used the printer to make new parts for itself that further enhanced its own functionality—a kind of perpetual motion machine, no?

than the opinions of later twentieth-century educators. That is, until he considered college applications. That's when things went sideways.

To consider a college for engineering, Lindhoff paused and thought. Surprisingly, he stumbled upon a storehouse of painful memories from his school days: a hodgepodge of reprimands, recriminations, under-performances, and flat-out failures. All the experiences Lindhoff for years branded as irrelevant and cast off—it turned out all that crap had been recorded and saved in memory. And for some reason, now, something went into his head and spliced together all the scenes of inferiority and I-told-you-so moments into a scathing sizzle reel. The loop, played on a screen visible only to Lindhoff's mind's eye, induced a dump of adrenaline that chased away every feeling except fear. Eventually even that evaporated, and all that remained was a chalky residue: inadequacy.

To his credit, Lindhoff did not flee from his self-inflicted shot of doubt. It would have been easy to do. He could have slinked from the fight completely and just written himself off as a screwup, something that every teacher from second grade onward would have endorsed. But he didn't. He could have deflected the issue by a devaluation of engineering schools as institutions of the privileged elite, and then embraced something more working-class, like welding. He didn't go for that either. Instead, in his first act of true bravery, invisible though it was to the world, Lindhoff managed to swallow fear whole: he decided to shoot straight at the target. Such was the magnitude of Lindhoff's love for mechanical expression.

Lindhoff gave himself permission to imagine a college career as an engineering student and a small miracle occurred: reality, in the form of the conjecture—"Maybe I should study for the SAT," or something to that effect. For the first time in his life, free time was freely given to a most improbable pursuit: *practice* exams. To stoop this low—such was the magnitude of Lindhoff's love for mechanical expression.

Then a second miracle occurred: Lindhoff discovered he was a math prodigy. The test questions proved a piece of cake, far simpler than deciphering virgin motherboards. His talent was innate but hitherto unknown—a masterpiece squirreled in a dusty attic, nonexistent until decluttered. Lindhoff put up a mammoth math subscore, and Carnegie-Mellon or Cal Tech seemed within reach.

Armed with scores and dreams, Lindhoff approached his father, a man whose career as a bookkeeper might have predicted a hearty attaboy slap on the back. Not so. The family wasn't wealthy, and Lindhoff the elder had pressures the son didn't appreciate—pressures middle-class fathers know all too well. His simple two-word response to his son's proposal for an A-tier college crushed the boy's spirit.

"Sounds expensive."

The parsimony was rich with implication; in particular that Lindhoff ought to recalibrate his sights onto a local community college. Which he did, since life is mostly unfair.[3]

———————•———————

Some twenty years later, the referral came from Dr. C., a psychoanalyst whom I'd shared a few cases with previously. She knew I had an interest in addictions, and further, my willingness to return her calls set me apart from other psychiatrists. These two proclivities could help her, and what Dr. C. needed was help. At a recent session, Lindhoff mentioned that he just spent an entire business trip in Los Angeles shooting heroin. However she pictured Lindhoff injecting himself,[4] the vision horrified the urbane Dr. C. She referred him to me reflexively, grateful to share the case with someone who spoke at length with patients who took great risks with special molecules. Together, the two of us would form the modern couple of mental health treatment— she the therapist and I the medication consultant.[5]

As he entered my office, there was nothing to Lindhoff's appearance that suggested he was an experienced user of intravenous heroin, known in some circles as a junkie. Dressed in a plaid Oxford shirt, absent a tie and

———————————————

3   Lindhoff eventually earned a four-year degree, but it wasn't in engineering.

4   The end of a tourniquet gripped in clenched teeth was one stock image.

5   How did this marriage form? Simple: via magnetic attraction. Over the past several decades, the number of non-MD psychotherapists has exploded. They cannot prescribe medications, but they treat a helluva lot of patients who need them.

unbuttoned at the neck, with casual slacks and standard-stock shoes, he could walk among the crowd of any American city, invisible.[6]

Owing to nerves, a lack of preparation, or maybe to never having taken a class on how to present a psychiatric history, Lindhoff began the consultation in scattered fashion. He sent me to ricochet around a landscape of depressive episodes, drug use episodes, and medication trials. Fortunately, I had taken some classes, and so we began again, methodically.

Depressive episodes seemed clear. When in their grip, Lindhoff wanted to retreat; and if the opportunity availed itself, he would simply stay in bed. Everything dialed down: energy, pleasure, motivation, thinking itself. Everything except melancholy—that ratcheted up and stuck to him like a pruritic rash. As much as he longed to lie still and be left alone when afflicted, Lindhoff was forced to push through and engage. He had a job, and a wife, and children who expected things from him. But, boy, was it a feat to act, to even move at times.

Not surprisingly, when depressed, Lindhoff felt he did a poor job of it at work, although definitive evidence was scant. His last review was not alarming, unless you found a mediocre review alarming. Though pasted over by depression, Lindhoff still had a personality under it all, and it turns out he was not the slacker type by temperament. Under ordinary circumstances Lindhoff would have overperformed

6   It makes you wonder how many other junkies are in the crowd.

at the job, but often he just didn't have the juice. That only made matters worse.

The situation at home was more obviously compromised. During the workweek, when Lindhoff returned from the office with his batteries tapped out, he could get away with a mindless pick at his dinner plate and then a burrow into bed. But that would not do on weekends—children and chores offered no cover. Nevertheless, the depressed Lindhoff could not conjure much motivation, and what little came forth was shunted to the job. So, at home, he chronically failed to deliver and played the part of a deadbeat. His wife was not happy. That only made matters worse.

These episodes of listless depression had blindsided Lindhoff since adolescence. Some bled into each other, separated by intervals of marginal improvement that could hardly be called acceptable. When you added these intervals of lousy existence to the mix, who's to say when Lindhoff *wasn't* under the spell of depression? His parents must have noticed something amiss because they sent him to a psychiatrist when still a teen. I counted at least twelve medication trials since then, over a period of twenty years, none memorable for inciting anything good.

The substance use history only added complexity. Lindhoff had self-administered quite an array of street drugs over the past two-dozen years. The breadth of his palette—cocaine, tranquilizers, opioids, alcohol, marijuana, psychedelics, and dissociatives—was impressive. And Lindhoff didn't just sip at these disparate drugs when happenstance brought them around. No, he sought and drank deeply of them *all*, and for long periods. He had his favorite partners of course, but at the same time, in a pinch, Lindhoff would go to the dance with whoever was in town. The guy simply loved drugs.[7]

What sense to make of this history? Twenty-plus years of on-and-off[8] depressive symptoms intertwined with a panoply of street drugs. Which came first, the depression or the drugs? Were they related, as in the circumstance when drugs run out and cause a crash into depression? Or did the converse relation apply, when depression causes drug use in an effort to self-medicate? Or were they independent—depression for depression's sake, and drug use for the sake of getting high?

It was a mess to sort out. A time line would have been helpful, but who keeps such a record? And could it be trusted, anyway? Reconstructed time lines are notoriously prone to bias, and when drugs and depression are involved, two kinds of bias are typically seen. Drug users can tilt towards understanding their use through the lens of depression—drugs become justified weapons in the war against despair. Drug nonusers (family, friends, law enforcement) often stake out the other camp—drug use is about getting high—an irresponsible, selfish, and

---

7   We have a nontechnical term for this type of substance user, someone who will heartily partake of whatever drug is available. He is known as a garbagehead.

8   Mostly on.

reprehensible behavior.[9] We would have to move forward for now; I did have other patients scheduled.

We returned to recent events. Lindhoff told me about his trip to Los Angeles. Up until then he'd been clean from heroin for five years, but for some reason, on that flight to LAX, he was seized with an irresistible urge to shoot up. It might have been related to an uptick in depression. Lindhoff had stopped his antidepressant about a month before the trip. He was no fan of the medicines—antidepressants never helped his mood enough to warrant their side effects. But that didn't mean things couldn't get worse if he stopped them.[10]

Whatever the reason for his itch, the West Hollywood heroin returned a delightful scratch and, as a bonus, lifted his spirits enormously. Lindhoff had a full week freed from depression's chains. That was the fuzzy truth—when Lindhoff looked back at the LA trip, he saw that heroin delivered both euphoria *and* euthymia.[11] There was a glassy nostalgia in his eyes as he recounted the run, a look very similar to the reminiscence of a tryst with a skillful lover.

---

9   Clinicians should be agnostic here and not take either side exclusively, since one side will invariably be wrong some of the time. No one uses a drug of abuse for the same reason on every occasion. Human behavior is not that predictable. The challenge is to determine which explanation is in play for a particular situation. However, since *both* motives can coexist simultaneously, even this rational approach is fraught. Patients can self-medicate a negative emotional state *and* indulge a desire to get high *at the same time*. In fact, this dual motive occurs quite often. It creates a very fuzzy picture for anyone accustomed to high-resolution photography. Welcome to addiction psychiatry.

10   Patients, and even some therapists, are often surprised by this.

11   Euthymia is the technical term for a normal mood state.

Irrespective of our potential disagreements on whether, for him, heroin was friend or foe, the immediate problem for Lindhoff was that after a week shooting a few bundles of dope, his crash was apocalyptic. Not the writhing chills of a diarrheic cold turkey detox, but rather a freefall to a take-your-breath-away depressive paralysis. He was back in the pit.

Lindhoff was grateful to have saved some Cymbalta, the last man out from his recent antidepressant retreat. He crawled to his medicine cabinet, found the bottle, and gulped a capsule. That was a few weeks ago. Now he sat opposite me, the tale told, and a question: "What the hell do I do now?"

An excellent question. Lindhoff was a hair better with a couple weeks of medicine in him, so "Certainly stay on the Cymbalta" seemed a good initial response. The second recommendation, that Lindhoff abstain from all drugs and alcohol, was not contested. The payback from a week on heroin had hurt Lindhoff badly, and he wasn't about to wade into those waters again any time soon. As for a new idea to treat depression, that would take some thought. Lindhoff understood, and agreed I should coordinate with Dr. C.

———•———

A few days after the consultation, over a landline, Dr. C. reiterated her gratitude for our collaboration on the Lindhoff case. His heroin use rattled her, more than his depression, and she found Lindhoff's fascination with drugs unsettling. This was understandable; addicted patients were not a part of Dr. C.'s training. Notwithstanding that, after Los Angeles, she upped her visits with Lindhoff to twice a week, to increase support. That was very kind of her.

Meanwhile, our phone call made crystal clear that I was now the quarterback for Lindhoff's treatment, responsible for all significant decisions, medical and otherwise. I had the expertise, the experience, the connection to resources, and the sole ability to prescribe medication. So it made sense that I was the quarterback. Ironically though, when Dr. C. doubled her treatment frequency, Lindhoff became *less* available to see *me*.[12]

In time, Lindhoff came back for his follow-up. He was still smarting from the binge in LA; the mere mention of heroin induced a revulsion I could plainly see. Lindhoff's mood had seesawed on Cymbalta and was sometimes fairly decent, but one thing stayed steady: he harped on a lack of motivation, and it became clear this was a big problem, even when not depressed. He felt the effects at work and at home; the gears just wouldn't catch. Productivity suffered in the office and was nonexistent elsewhere. He could fake it pretty well when not in the pit, but Lindhoff yearned to do things naturally and effortlessly, to *want* to do things, as he imagined others could. To make matters worse, Lindhoff had just transferred to a new department and was already

12 You see the conundrum that occurs sometimes for psychiatrists who serve as "med backup" for therapists. I am the quarterback, and I come out to run the big play every so often, but I don't train with the team. Someone else does that.

behind the eight ball with added responsibilities. He pressed me for a more muscular pharmacology.

Spurred by this plea for help, I started to fiddle with Lindhoff's medications. Not for nothing, but a smarter person would have seen this as a fool's errand—just look at the results from two decades of previous efforts. Yeah, well, certain psychiatrists are known to stubbornly ignore history's lessons, and think their own grasp of pharmacology more nuanced than their predecessors. Although I don't often count myself in this cohort, at this moment, for Lindhoff, I went to the closet and found my jester's cap. I tried a bunch of stuff based on some clever theory: activation of dopaminergic motivational circuits. It's not important. It didn't work. They didn't help.[13]

I'll tell you what *was* important, though: the day Lindhoff showed up for his session with a wide, beatific smile. I knew instantly that something big had happened to him. We'd been sputtering through my fanciful med trials when Lindhoff took matters into his own hands. He researched the web and found a new dissociative[14] from a trusted source in Spain. The molecule was an indole derivative, hexa-methyl-indolamine,[15] and word on Reddit hailed HMI as the new "it" dissociative.

---

13 I should have known better.

14 The dissociatives are curious drugs that cause the body to temporarily separate from the whole as far as conscious awareness is concerned. To find this disconnected state euphoric is an acquired taste no doubt. The allure of the dissociative high has something to do with an uncanny calm that emerges when one isn't encumbered by a body. Who knew?

15 Hexa-methyl-indolamine (HMI) does not actually exist; it is a made-up chemical name. The actual compound Lindhoff took will not be disclosed.

Lindhoff was euphoric—well, oceanic was probably a better descriptor. He spoke of a vast openness that had overtaken his consciousness. It could be seen in the way he held his body at rest, perfectly at ease. It could be heard in the soothing timbre of his voice. It could be acknowledged in the transcendent content of his language. And then there was that smile—it was a stunner. You had to be there, but trust me when I tell you, I believed him. If you threw a saffron robe on the guy, I would've thought him a bodhisattva. Wow. I think that Spanish hexa-methylindolamine was mislabeled. This was like nothing I'd read in the textbooks about dissociatives.

Amazingly, Lindhoff had been like this for days, and had even gone to work. He dosed himself over the past weekend, while his wife was away with the kids. The effects I saw were actually down considerably from their peak. He had not hallucinated at any time during the trip, it was all about openness. Oh, yeah, one more thing: naturally, the depression and amotivation were completely gone. He felt great, way better than great, and seemed to be functioning just fine.

I had to admit the Spanish molecule was impressive, but it was to a fault. The intensity of the drug's effect made it impractical for any kind of sustained use. Lindhoff must have seen that; it was obvious. He could not realistically expect Spain to solve his problems.

Of course, Lindhoff's little experiment also showed me maybe I was naïve to have trusted him to keep our agreement on abstinence. Fair enough. They say substance abusers tell everyone a different bit of the truth, but no one the whole truth. I think that's true, but it's not because they're substance abusers. *No one* tells anyone the whole truth, about anything.[16] Regardless, this was not the time to reprimand Lindhoff on his violation—I doubt it would have penetrated his rapture.

Lindhoff had been worn down by amotivation and depression, I get it. Still, when he ordered the hexa-methyl-indolamine, did he envision it as a medicine to *remedy* these symptoms or an intoxicant to *replace* them? Fuzzy, right? My bet was both, but I would have to wait for Lindhoff to fully clear, like a common drunk in the tank, before any discussion. That could take days, it seemed. Lindhoff had not yet visited Dr. C. this week—she hadn't had the pleasure of bathing in his aura. I didn't see "enlightenment" as a reason to hold Lindhoff any further so I sent him on his way to Dr. C., confident the truth about the weekend would simply follow him through the door.

———————•———————

Dr. C. dutifully called me after meeting with Lindhoff, and she had some blockbuster news. Apparently, Lindhoff's Spanish-induced openness persisted into their session and led him to come clean in a most unexpected way. In addition to his recent ingestion of HMI, Lindhoff revealed that he'd been regularly injecting various other European and Asian substances for *years*—

16 Don't let them fool you.

research chemicals on no one's watch list, neither illegal nor detectable. It was enough to make the head spin.[17]

Lindhoff was whisked away to rehab after the revelation. I never did have my talk about why he pulled the trigger on the Spanish magic powder. Everyone needed a break to reassess the situation, not the least of whom must have been Lindhoff's wife. Whatever she thought she knew of his drug exploits, it was but the tip of the iceberg. And whatever her reaction, I imagined Lindhoff would welcome some time out of the house, out of her eyeshot.

The rehab kept him a month. They did not change the psych meds I prescribed. The rehab appeared to favor the view that Lindhoff used drugs primarily for their own sake, for the high, rather than to self-medicate. That could be a reasonable conclusion given the recent discovery of Lindhoff's multinational shenanigans.[18]

What the rehab did change was Lindhoff's psychological treatment. He returned home to a new team: an addiction-trained psychologist, an addiction-focused group, and an addiction-informed couple therapy. These clinicians and services were added onto Lindhoff's existing treatment with Dr. C., who now seemed distinctly like the odd doc out. But what was the rehab

---

17 Were it not for the Spanish molecule, Lindhoff would probably be keeping his secrets to this day. Even so, it didn't escape that, despite his drug-induced "openness," Lindhoff did not tell *me* about the chronic injection use, only Dr. C. Maybe she was the quarterback on some of the plays after all.

18 Perhaps my error was to underestimate the appetite of a garbagehead.

to do? Cut Dr. C. from the aftercare plan because she had no addiction chops? Lindhoff was her patient. That would be very bad for business.

I survived Lindhoff's treatment team re-org and continued to see him. Dr. C. either got the hint or got smart. When Lindhoff told her he was overextended with the new therapists, she graciously stepped aside.

Over the next six months the treatment shifted. It became one hundred percent about the therapies, now run by properly trained professionals who, however, weren't interested a whit in collaboration. My phone did not ring. I saw Lindhoff infrequently. The meds weren't changing, so why come in to see an expensive addiction psychiatrist? Lindhoff appeared to buy into the new model. He said he was finally abstinent from exotic drugs, as required by his therapists to stay in treatment. He felt reasonably well. His main complaint was boredom, but he wasn't pushing for any medication adjustments. The patient was improved, and I was back on the sidelines.

———•———

This halcyon picture ended the day I got a call from Lindhoff's wife, Annie, her first to me. Something seemed off, and she wanted a quick chat. Mrs. L. was remarkably calm on the phone as she described her husband's psychosis. I hadn't ever met Annie, so I wasn't sure whether her manner represented a self-possessed character or was the kind of no-big-deal stance we all take at times when confronted with something we desperately hope is nothing.

Lindhoff had stopped sleeping and spoke of new powers to bring love into the world and change the course of history. I opined that this was not typically seen in garden-variety insomnia and sounded instead like the Spanish molecule on overdrive. Given the delusion, and the unpredictable nature of abrupt-onset deities, I directed Annie to get her spouse to the local emergency room by whatever means necessary. She hesitated, as we all do at times when confronted with something we desperately hope is nothing. To reassure her, I reminded Annie that she knew her man—he had enough trouble getting off his ass to change a light bulb, let alone the destiny of humankind. She agreed. As did the psych ER.

When the three of us met a few weeks later, after his discharge from the inpatient psychiatric unit, the first thing I did was toss Lindhoff's new diagnosis of bipolar disorder in the garbage. The hospital took his symptoms literally, and neglected the power of the Spanish molecule to mimic euphoric mania. Without powerful, mood-altering drugs on board, Lindhoff could muster about as much euphoria as a brick. He was not bipolar.

Lindhoff was cagey about why he revisited HMI after months of stability with the new therapists.[19] The origin of his psychosis was less ambiguous. The come-down from a couple generous hits of HMI led to depressive

19 My bet was he got fed up with boredom.

symptoms that Lindhoff was terrified would repeat the calamity of the West Hollywood heroin. So, he doubled down with even more generous hits. That shot him out of depression all right, with panache, and he became a God for a few days. A week of inpatient later, marinated with antipsychotics and cleared of the Spanish indole, and he was back on terra firma.

If I expected contrition, I was to be disappointed. How about a new agenda instead? Lindhoff was nothing if not resourceful when it came to considering chemicals to goose his synaptic traffic. He took full advantage of his time on the psych ward—what better place to do street research? He threw me a curve.

"Doc, I want to try ketamine."[20]

"Ketamine?"

"Yes, ketamine. There's something to the dissociatives. I think this can help my mood."

"Yes, there is certainly something to the dissociatives. They make you psychotic."

"C'mon, Doc. I'll be monitored."

He had a point. Ketamine would be a safer way to try a dissociative, as long as he didn't freelance more Spanish excursions on top of it. Could there be a way for Lindhoff to harness the antidepressant effect of dissociatives—without inducing enlightenment or frank psychosis? Ketamine was the best chance. And anyway,

---

20 Ketamine is a dissociative anesthetic that has been used to treat depression. It is also a club drug of abuse. Recently the FDA approved a version of ketamine for treatment-resistant depression.

by now, I doubted Lindhoff could resist the Spanish molecule without a robust alternative.

"Sure, why not?"

I made the requisite referrals to the modern doctors who mix and administer ketamine.[21] Ironically, the potion was delivered via a forty-five minute intravenous infusion that by all accounts was pleasantly trippy, when accompanied by the right music. Nice. Lindhoff now got his dissociative high sanctioned by Psychiatry, with soundtrack sanctioned by Tangerine Dream. Wouldn't you know it though, with his luck, ketamine was a complete bust as an antidepressant. No benefit. It simply did not move the needle. Lindhoff was foiled. Shoulders drooped, he went back to my meds, the usual suspects.

There ensued a few months of peace and quiet when I didn't hear a peep from Lindhoff. I returned to the rest of my practice—patients in trouble with whiskey, painkillers, weed, etc. Drugs people had heard of, and had a sense of. Familiar territory. It was a relief to be back in my comfort zone, curled up near the fire in a favorite cardigan, maybe with a glass of Calvados if it happened to be Christmas Eve.[22]

———•———

But it's hard to keep the peace. Lindhoff eventually reached out with a text.

---

21 They will likely inherit the future of psychiatry.
22 Metaphorically speaking.

> Doc, can we meet next week? I'd like to share some research with you. I think it will be interesting for both of us. I'll be bringing Annie along. It's good news.

Damn if he wasn't back at it with the Spanish molecule.

They came in, and Lindhoff made his case. After the disappointment with ketamine, Lindhoff settled back into his malcontented baseline. He took my meds, but the best they could do was offer shitty respite. I had invited Lindhoff to shelter under my umbrella, but there wasn't enough room for him so he stood half out in the rain, and got half soaked. This would not do. Ever the problem-solver,[23] but with few tools left in the shed, Lindhoff turned again to the Spanish molecule. Was it possible to walk a fine line with the potent Catalonian powder—up to the border of salvation but not into the realm of psychosis? Lindhoff, weary to swim upstream for every little thing, was up to the challenge.

Undeterred by the trivial risks of psychosis, hospitalization, divorce, and unemployment, Lindhoff got himself a chemist's scale and started experimenting with precise doses of HMI. Today he brought Annie in to vouch for his results. When consumed at fifteen milligrams every four days, HMI produced one hour of dissociative euphoria without delusions, followed

---

23 Remember Lindhoff was an engineer at heart.

by four days of normal mood and motivation. Annie confirmed the absence of psychosis, and the absence of procrastination. Her husband had become more productive, more functional, and more pleasant to live with. I could see Annie was happy with her new man.

"Very well then, you're right. It's an interesting result. And I can see why you'd want to keep it going. But you don't need me for that. You can do this on your own."

Lindhoff frowned. "No, I want to keep seeing you. I don't want to come off your meds. I don't know what would happen. I'd like to keep taking the HMI on top of your regimen. But we want you to stay involved. We want you to manage the treatment."

It was my turn to frown. "You want me to manage the treatment? The treatment that now includes fifteen milligrams of a white powder from Spain? A powder that came to you with no clinical data, no safety data, no purity data, and no data to confirm that it is actually hexa-methyl-indolamine, whatever that even is. The only thing we know for sure about that powder is that it can cause psychosis. Is that the treatment you want me to manage?"

"Doc, I've been using HMI for a while now. I'm well below the psychotic dose threshold. Annie can attest to that. She's been involved in every aspect of this new protocol. I measure it out in front of her every four or five days. We speak constantly. I answer all her questions. After that first hour, I'm good. Doc, my mood is finally good. Not crazy with the openness and love, just normal, neutral. And I'm not dragging myself through everything. I just get up and do it. Doc, I'm not euphoric, not even close. I'm just good. Doc, I'm *good*. And I want to stay there."

A silence descended on the three of us.

How could I begrudge Lindhoff his antics with the Spanish molecule? His brain didn't work right, and he wanted it fixed. What had Psychiatry offered him? Feeble medicines with nagging side effects. And Addiction Psychiatry's recipe? More feeble medicines *and* a prohibition on drugs, because *maybe* they were part of the problem. We couldn't even be sure, the picture is so complicated.[24]

Lindhoff went awfully far in search of his own solution. And I had to ask myself, whether from drugs or depression, if it were *my* fate to have never really felt right in my own skin, how far would *I* go to feel better? How far would anyone go? Pretty damn far, many of us.

I looked over to Annie. She had no drug history; she was an accountant. Solid head on her shoulders. Yeoman's job raising kids while working full time. She nodded back at me gently, nothing dramatic, just a quiet confirmation of her husband's account. I trusted her. Lindhoff *was* in fact better these weeks on HMI— better in all the ways that mattered to him, and to her. The Spanish molecule was about Annie, too, and her

---

24 Ketamine is an excellent case in point: club drug for years, now vanguard for the treatment of depression.

children. They were all on a chain gang, working the same craggy road for years, now with a glimmer of hope in the form of a foreign synthetic chemical.

Years ago a teacher summarized addiction for me in a single glib statement: "People do what they wanna do."[25] Lindhoff would continue to use the Spanish molecule whatever I decided. The choice for me was whether to stay on the case despite the uncertainty or cut him loose *because* of the uncertainty.

"Both of you are prepared to accept the risks of this hexa-methyl-indolamine: unknown toxicity to organ systems, the possibility of future psychotic episodes, or other brain dysfunction, the unknown long-term effects? This is all uncharted territory."

"We do," they vowed in unison.

Oh, hell…all right. Somebody's got to make sure he doesn't make a mess of it. Who's that going to be?

"The only way I'd consider staying involved is if you agree to a few things. You've got to find a lab to verify the chemical composition of the powder and its purity. We do a literature search of the compound and contact anyone who's studied it. You will get bloodwork every three months to track basic labs. Also, I'm not happy with even an hour of dissociation. I want you to drop the dose to three milligrams. You can take that every day as long as it causes no euphoria or dissociation. Oh, and one more thing, at

---

25 She undersold herself—this insight applies to human behavior in general.

the first hint of any symptom approaching psychosis, we shut down the experiment."

"Agreed, no problem." Lindhoff and Annie relaxed. "Thank you."

Yeah, you're welcome.

Lindhoff did his due diligence. The Spanish molecule was indeed confirmed to be hexa-methyl-indolamine. There were a few references to HMI in the literature, but only on the chemistry, nothing about clinical use in humans. Lindhoff discovered that four milligrams per day produced no intoxication effects. His labs were normal. Psychiatrically, Lindhoff presented a clean sheet: stable mood, little procrastination, improved social relationships, abstinence from other drugs, enviable sense of well-being. No complaints.

We cruised like this with no turbulence for months. Lindhoff couldn't remember when he'd felt and functioned this well for this long. The Spanish molecule had changed the game. I suggested we plan for a one-year trial of HMI, and then taper off to see if the response held.[26] I thought about writing up Lindhoff's case for publication; maybe we were on to the next ketamine!

Dammit when circumstances get in the way of exciting plans.

I was studying at home for the addiction psychiatry re-credentialing exam[27] when I got a text from Lindhoff.

---

26 I was approaching HMI as I would any traditional antidepressant.
27 I kid you not.

The exchange went as follows:

> Hi Dr. M. The experiment has been terminated (abruptly and without apparent repercussions) due to a series of unfortunate events. Assume you'd advise to continue with my regular medications as I'm doing. I'll fill you in when we next meet unless you'd like to touch base sooner.

> Of course I'm curious.

> In a nutshell, I was released from jail and part of the terms of my freedom are that I remain free of drugs.

> What was the offense?

> Possession of firearms (locked away securely in my home) without a permit. Police ended up in my house due to 911 call of medical nature related to substance abuse.

> A very unfortunate tale. We should meet.

Lindhoff came in alone and didn't look any worse for wear. He launched his narrative posthaste. The story deserved a bowl of popcorn had I known, but I kept none in the office. On the day in question, Lindhoff got high, and had taken too big a hit. He was in the kitchen when he felt the rush about to overtake him, and he clumsily lowered himself to the floor before full unconsciousness set in. Annie discovered him there out cold, and knowing enough to know she couldn't possibly know what he took, called 911.

Flat on his back, Lindhoff came to in his kitchen, staring up at a crowd of EMS techs and police officers. He was mighty groggy. The techs peppered him with questions as he slowly cleared. After they established that orientation to person, place, and time was intact, the techs moved on to the matter of how Lindhoff arrived on the kitchen floor unconscious. Lindhoff was adept at keeping secrets, but believe it or not, it wasn't his nature to lie at direct questions. That trait, coupled with the stupor he found himself in, and Lindhoff started to sing like a canary.

As Lindhoff struggled to explain his relationship with the Spanish molecule, one police officer peeled off the group and began to meander around the first floor of Lindhoff's home. In the living room he took notice of a small wooden box. It wasn't the grain, or finish, or artistry that caught his eye—the object was so plain as to guarantee no attention at a yard sale. No, it was the shape of the container. The officer had seen elongated, narrow wooden boxes like that before. They were the perfect size to hold an optical sight for a rifle.

The officer did not touch the box. He returned to the kitchen, found the spot he vacated a few minutes prior, got into a crouch, and asked Lindhoff the question that would change things for a while.

"Sir, do you own any firearms?"

By now Lindhoff had cleared enough to sit up. Under the circumstances, the officer's question seemed a colossal non sequitur, but Lindhoff was on a roll with the truth, and so it just came out. Yes, he responded. In fact, he owned several firearms, including long guns, handguns, and one automatic rifle.

Then came the question that would really change things for a while.

"Sir, are these weapons registered?"

Ah, that *was* an issue, non sequitur or not. The answer was no, and to jump ahead a little, that led Lindhoff to jail instead of an emergency room. It took his lawyer a week to get him out on bail. I hear that's par for the course when the charge is felony possession of a *machine gun*, registered or not.

Lindhoff took a pause in his recitation, and I thought it a good moment to close my mouth. It took awhile longer to formulate thoughts, but they eventually came.

"You had all these firearms? Why?"

It was about assembly, stupid—his old hobby, to build things. Back in the day, Lindhoff discovered he could fabricate guns. They weren't actually that hard to build, certainly less so than the 3-D printer. Of course, Lindhoff loved a challenge, and he got caught up in pushing the envelope. Handguns led to rifles, which led to the machine gun. The irony was, after shooting them once or twice to confirm they worked, Lindhoff lost interest. He disassembled the weapons and locked them away. That was years ago. He didn't tell me about the guns because he had forgotten about them. There never was a thought of registration because he never expected to use the weapons again.

The State saw it differently. He was on the hook for up to five years in jail.[28]

"And the HMI? You took a mega-dose that day? Why?"

"No, I didn't take HMI, not any more than usual anyway. A couple weeks ago I went on the Spanish website to order some more for the rest of the year. I noticed a new synthetic cannabinoid[29] and decided to get some as a little treat for myself. *That's* what I took that morning, the synthetic weed. I took the tiniest hit, but it knocked me on my ass."

No kidding, Avogadro. That's what happens when you practice chemistry without a license.

Great—*another* fucking Spanish molecule.

---

28 Lindhoff was ultimately able to plead to a lower charge after a year of wrangling.

29 Synthetic marijuana, far more powerful than the natural plant.

POSTSCRIPT

Over the years, I've seen many addicted patients convinced that the drug they abuse is the only thing that can save them from depression, or some other infirmity. Unfortunately, most are doomed to fail "controlled use" for "medicinal purposes," because addiction doesn't condone controlled use. Loss of control is addiction's *sine qua non*. It is the wild horse.

Still, occasionally there is success. Some addicted individuals *can* modulate their use for an adaptive advantage. I suspect most of these instances never present for treatment and remain invisible to Medicine. Why should they present to a doctor? If the drug is working... it ain't broke, so why fix it?

Was Lindhoff in this category? He *did* eventually return to daily use of four milligrams of HMI, after the legal heat cooled. Had Lindhoff discovered the right dose to sit in the Spanish molecule's sweet spot, and thereby end his decades-long quest for sustained euthymia? And was he able to override the pull for reckless, unbridled use?

In other words, did Lindhoff tame the wild horse??[30]

---

30 YES!!

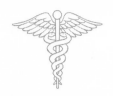

TUNA AU POIVRE

---

*The psychiatrist's best teacher, of course, is the patient. That should be gift enough, especially when you consider that the psychiatrist also gets **paid** for being taught. Yet some patients have an uncanny spirit of generosity and give more on top of this.*

From my experience, the more ill the patient—the more remarkable the gift.

RICHIE COULD'VE BEEN Bourdain, long before Bourdain, if he had the capacity to put the word to paper. I had no idea if the man could write; but, boy, could he spin a good yarn one on one. A real raconteur, that one. Smooth as silk. I envied his skills.

Looks helped—Richie had a Brad Pitt vibe. Early Pitt. Very early. *A River Runs Through It* early. The rest of the package, self-deprecation and the savage truth, put him up there with the best of the Soviet satirists.

He worked IT for a suite of downtown restaurants. Hell, for all I knew he might've hung out with Bourdain at *Les Halles* before Kitchen Confidential hit the charts. I wouldn't have been surprised.

I wish I remembered more details of Richie's life, but the fact is our treatment had a specific focus that often precluded discretionary chit-chat. He came to see me for one thing and one thing only: outpatient detox from heroin. From a physician's perspective, this service was typically concerned with detailed, no-nonsense evaluations of meaningful human physiology.

Despite this clear clinical agenda, it was Richie's preference to regale me with the latest high jinks perpetrated in his client kitchens. Propped up with massive doses of alcohol and cocaine, the boys on the line committed hilarious and disgusting atrocities to the plate. Richie was a keen observer of the human condition, of what the prospect of having to make rent could do to some people. Honestly though, Richie knew when he met a mark he could manipulate. The troubadour act was meant to defend against any genuine discussion of *his own* human mis-condition. Any talk of treatment after detox and Richie would launch into one his hundred tales, like the time crackhead Squeegee nearly severed Skinny's pinky in a ratatouille prep mishap. A downright Decameron, he was.

Richie's heroin addiction fit right into the mayhem of the kitchen. He would come to me when the burden of shooting a bundle of dope a day got too heavy. This was in the 1990s, pre-Suboxone, when heroin detox involved prescribing a cocktail of non-opioid meds to blunt the intensity of withdrawal: clonidine for chills, valium for anxiety, trazodone for sleep, among other things. I gave the meds out myself. Bought 'em in bulk from Hank Schein and kept them in my top drawer. Counted out enough to make it to the next appointment, put them in an envelope, and wrote the directions on the front. I found this procedure improved outcome. Really couldn't expect a dopesick addict to wait for a bunch of prescriptions at Duane Reade.

I did a good enough job with Richie to help him get over the hump. Then, he'd disappear. No goodbye, no nothing. Just stopped showing up—until the next jam. I detoxed him three times in total. Never saw him for more than two weeks in a row, though. In cases like this, I often wonder whether I'm more a cutman for a boxer.

To be completely fair, Richie also had a drinking problem, but this apparently never bothered him. For the third detox, he showed up in heroin withdrawal *and* drunk. He had been gifted a cache of Hennessy. No problem. We doubled down and did a double detox. Every session had the same drill: blood pressure, pulse, pupillary size, symptom checklist, pill count, new set of pill envelopes, and new tales of culinary misadventures. He told me the alcohol was coming down.

About two weeks into this stint, Richie called me to say he was coming uptown and might be a little late. He showed up absolutely stinking drunk, with a plain brown shopping bag in tow. The reek of booze filled the office and, as he staggered into the couch, I sat dumbfounded and re-breathed his fetid, exhaled alcohol. After his best effort to sit upright, Richie said he brought me some lunch and began to clumsily unpack the bag. Out came a set of cutlery wrapped in a linen serviette. Next came a large, clear plastic takeout container that housed a professionally cooked serving for one of wild rice, broccoli rabe, and the fattest piece of tuna au poivre I had even seen. The fish was completely encased in a peppercorn embossment, Tellicherry by the look of it.

Finally, with a third tremulous descent into the bag, a bottle of Tuscan merlot emerged.

Richie had taxied up from a well-known restaurant whose reservations were difficult to secure. He vouched for the cleanliness of the repast and insisted I eat it right then and there, in front of him. He did not bring any nourishment for himself. I had to think quickly here—I was afraid breathing the vapor from his lungs a bit longer might render me secondarily intoxicated.

Well, it *was* lunchtime, and we are taught that there *are* exceptions to the rule that psychiatrists shouldn't accept gifts. The meal would lose any remaining warmth without rapid, decisive action. There was also Richie's disappointment to think of.

I began to unfold the beige, linen serviette, itself as fine as a 300-count Egyptian cotton coverlet. The cutlery within had noticeable heft. In addition to the oversized fork and spoon, Richie had included an impressively large, wooden-handled steak knife that could've come straight out of Peter Luger's.

Draping the serviette across my lap, I cracked open the takeout container. Richie encouraged me to uncork the wine; he had personally chosen the bottle to pair with the tuna. I respectfully declined, citing afternoon consultations. Richie bowed his head deeply and, with an Elizabethan flourish, gestured an arm forward.

I addressed the fare. First, the wild rice. The soft, pale grains were bespeckled with a moderate density of spindle-shaped, jet black cousins. They added a pleasant crunch to the textural experience, without undue effort. It did not escape me that the rice had taken up a salty French bouillon. Subtle.

Then, the broccoli rabe. Wilted to perfect submission, the stalks lay stacked in a heap, each adorned with a beckoning, understated, and unbruised floret. I speared one and bit off the blossom. The rabe's bitterness had not been fully neutralized by the chef's blanch. A gush of garlic butter, invisible to the eye, was easily detected. Exquisite.

Lastly, the tuna. The beast had the shape and thickness of a tenderloin medallion, and with the peppercorn crust it even looked the part. Finally, that magnificent knife had purpose. I grasped its handsome hilt and sliced a triangular morsel off the mother lode. Seared rare, of course. The sting of pepper spray was never so satisfying, assuaged in sequence by Dijon and burgundy vinegar, then blended all together within the succulence of the fish's creamy flesh. Sublime.

It was a culinary ecstasy, but I managed to hold onto good manners and only sampled a few mouthfuls of each element. I placed the regal leftovers on my desk, and then Richie announced he had a present for me.

"Another?"

Yes, he said, something that would last. He reached down to the bottom of the shopping bag and pulled out a second folded serviette. One or two flaps were pulled back, and there they were: three more steak knives. He wanted me to have a proper set.

"Enjoy them, Doc, and don't neglect the merlot."

Richie then fled as he arrived, full of surprises and unanswered questions. The heroin detox was apparently near completion; he left with no new med packets. As for alcohol, that was clearly a work in progress, even if only in my mind. About a week or two later, with no further word from Richie, I realized he was finished with me, for now. I'd have to wait until the next detox.

As it turned out I would never see Richie again; our last session together was that escapade with the poivre. But I wasn't done with him. I had those steak knives, and I got into the habit of using them as my daily cutlery. They became the default knife at my table, and as such the association to Richie faded over time. Every once in a while though, for unknown reasons, as I gathered them from the knife drawer, I would be thrust back to the memory of Richie and the tuna au poivre. At those moments I imagined he was out there somewhere in a high-end kitchen, probably shooting dope, wryly observing the mischief of the men on the line, each in his own way just trying to hang on.

Somewhere deep in Richie's brain, deeper than stories can penetrate, I'm pretty sure Richie knew he was just hanging on too.

POSTSCRIPT

The funny thing was, those restaurant-grade knives weren't as sturdy as they seemed. After some time, maybe a couple of years, the wood started to separate, and the handles became loose. With no obvious mechanism to tighten them, one by one they had to be retired. When I got down to two knives, in an effort to slow the decline, I stopped the daily use and reserved the pair for extra-special meals, like when a respectable Porterhouse made an appearance.

Five years after the tuna, I got a call from Nora, who told me she was Richie's ex-girlfriend. She wanted to come in for her own consultation. Nora had a nagging problem—she became suicidal the week before every period. Hey, any friend of Richie's…

During her consultation, it became clear Nora had been carrying my number for a while. When she told me Richie had died of a heroin overdose the year prior, she cried softly. Disbelief can be a useful reaction to loss. It allowed me to help Nora that day.

I was down to one steak knife by then. After the meeting with Nora, it became *my* knife, for use only by *me*, just a couple of times a year on the highest of holidays.

Eventually, even that was too much.

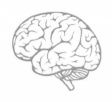

CASE EIGHT

WAITING FOR THE MAN

There is a tradition in Medicine that will make sense to you, namely that a physician ought endeavor to explain a patient's presentation as completely as possible with the fewest diagnoses, ideally just one. Doctors like certainty.

Occasionally though, psychiatric cases are so complex, one would need to be a contortionist to make everything fit under one diagnosis.

In those circumstances, psychiatrists should heed a lesson from rocket scientists, the smartest of whom know the difference between a complex equation on paper and flammable fuel in the tank.

EVAN WAS WHAT is known in the business as a diagnostic dilemma. It wasn't for a lack of effort. Many clinicians had taken a crack at his diagnosis. Each seemed a blind man with an elephant, carefully describing a small part of the whole. Several had produced lengthy reports, which Evan provided me at the start of our treatment together. The thickness of a psychiatric patient's chart is a good measure of past and future difficulty, and before we even started, Evan's chart was thicker than patients' I'd worked with for fifteen years.

I could see why Evan befuddled the clinicians before me. He was born and raised in comfortable privilege on Central Park West, with a pretty view above the treetops. He attended an exclusive private school, an exclusive boarding school, and an exclusive Ivy League college. He did reasonably well in academics, played some sports, and graduated on time.

That said, by college, blemishes in behavior coalesced into a blotch that required attention. Fits of anger grew ugly and culminated in the occasional pummeling of a roommate. Bouts of depression multiplied, with longer and longer periods of self-imposed exile. Rare but startling catatonia—spells of nonresponsive staring—reliably frightened family and friends alike.

Evan started to consult with experts. As he shared the details of his *inner* life, blemishes in *thought* joined their behavioral counterparts, and created an uncertain mental landscape. No one was able to arrive at a diagnosis that explained all Evan was capable of, internally and externally. The earliest report in my dossier, conducted during his freshman year at college, suggested emerging schizophrenia, then two sentences later emphatically clarified that Evan did "**not**" meet criteria for "**current**" schizophrenia. A subsequent evaluator puzzled over Evan's anger and violent fantasies, and, at a loss for the proper clinical nomenclature, started his summary with the colloquial "a seriously troubled young man." That would turn out to be as good a diagnosis as any.

Taken together, the records were more useful as Rorschach tests on the therapists themselves, rather than as clinical navigation tools. What did the evaluators see in Evan the inkblot? Anger towards women as a reaction to an icy, unfeeling mother? Grandiose fantasies of cultural fame as a solution to the problem of a demanding, workaholic father? An anxious and insecure man who longed for intimacy but saw human connection as a destructive force, and therefore defaulted to the paranoid position? A depressive—a legacy of his forebears—with coping skills that tended towards the magical? Take your pick, but realize you will disclose your bias in doing so.

By the time he got to me Evan had a serious cocaine dependence that, while insufficient to explain the fullness of the man, needed urgent attention. He was no treatment rookie; Evan had been through it all: inpatient, outpatient, individual, 12-step, sober living, sober coaching, CBT, DBT, meditation, psychodrama, and numerous medication trials, to name a few modalities.

Many patients who chronically relapse despite all this effort grow weary of expensive multimodal treatment. They yearn for a simpler sober life and can grow resentful towards the bloated entourage of addiction providers. They begin to think "less is more," which is often correct in matters of photography composition, but not necessarily so in matters of human disease. As a logical consequence to this kind of paradigm shift, patients often opt to shrink their treatment footprint. Private practice addiction psychiatrists, with discreet and comfortable offices in nice parts of town, can be easily incorporated into these minimalist fantasies. Enter Evan.

I want to make clear that it took several years to appreciate the breadth and depth of Evan's issues. At the initial visit, however, the focus was rather narrow and straightforward. Evan had relapsed onto two grams of pulverized cocaine, which, to administer, he snorted methodically up each nostril. The crystalline drug was prepared, through meticulous mincing with a single-edge razor blade, to form powdery lines of medium-fine talc. This practice increased the surface area of the contraband considerably. A vigorous insufflation, via any of a number of cylindrical fabrications placed into the nostril, would spray a high-velocity shower of tiny particles deep into the naso-pharynx, the curved tunnel that connects the nose to the throat. In this way, thousands of specks of cocaine dust would slam into the soft, moist surface of that conduit, where they would adhere, dissolve, and be taken in by the highly absorbent lining. Ultimately, individual cocaine molecules would find their way into the bloodstream and shoot up to the brain, where the machinery of euphoria awaited the illicit fuel.

Evan dosed his two grams in a succession of lines until his entire supply was finished, typically from about 8 p.m. to 5 a.m. He watched pornography on his computer and compulsively masturbated for most of that time. Somehow, after these festive nights with scant sleep, Evan would still manage to drag himself to work. That couldn't have been a fun day at the office. He'd crash early that evening and take the next day to replenish whatever metabolites were ravaged by the cocaine storm that had passed through his brain. On day three, towards the end of his shift, forces would conspire, and he'd get an urge to order up another two grams, which he would, and then have at it again all night long. This triplet pattern had gone on nearly three weeks now, and Evan was beginning to fray at the edges.

He had come in with the icy mother, who seemed to know more than any mother should about her adult son's private life. Whatever they hoped from an office-based approach with a solo practitioner, the fact remained that I was not a magician, or even a chiropractor, and so I had nothing to offer beyond the usual technologies for the treatment of cocaine addiction. I saw the disappointment in the mother's face.

I worked with Evan for several years. I fear a synopsis of that effort would bore in its repetition and technical minutia—the frequent cajoling to enter a more intensive group program, entreaties to stay connected to 12-step meetings and sponsors, the scramble to try to limit access to cash, the shifting landscape caused by erratic compliance to prescribed medications, and on and on. I suppress a yawn just writing about this.

The reader may not take for granted my assurance that less is more when it comes to the clinical description of Evan's treatment. What about the diagnostic dilemma, you might question? What role did it play in the relative success or failure in treating the cocaine addiction? Well, funny you should ask. Since I came to no better diagnostic impression than "a seriously troubled young man," I really have no idea, but I'm sure it didn't help.

I know this will not be good enough for many of you who have faithfully read my other case reports. As you are aware, I hope, my debt to your loyalty goes hand in hand with a constitutional aversion to disappoint.

Therefore, despite my inability to untangle the knotty Mr. Evan, let me share three small vignettes to both sate your interest in case material and reward your investment to have trudged this far in the essay.

SMALL VIGNETTE ONE

I risk disappointment at the outset since you will see our first offering is not a vignette at all. It is merely a few notations.

To sit with Evan would bring anyone into contact with the inscrutable. I didn't see the anger so much, or hear about the violent fantasies directly. My examination of the elephant bespoke of a vast emptiness to Evan's inner experience. Many examples of this surfaced in our discussions, but the time I realized his apartment contained no book or wall furnishing whatsoever will suffice as metaphor.

The emptiness was frightening, no more so than when others intruded into it. I remember the realization of what I was up against when Evan told me about the time he went to dinner with a friend from AA. He got so uncomfortable at that outing that he left his seat mid-meal, then left the restaurant, then took the subway home to his apartment. He never called the friend later to explain his actions. Evan knew something was terribly wrong with this kind of behavior, but I never did find a way to change his experience of human beings.

SMALL VIGNETTE TWO

There came a time, during a particularly ferocious stretch of cocaine use, that I drew the counterintuitive conclusion that Evan was not, actually, addicted to cocaine. Not in a primary sense. His actual problem, I posited, was pornography.

The reader may suspect by now that I am more interested to ask a good question than to propose a good answer. In the former, as I've learned the hard way, I'm less likely to fall through a rotted floorboard. So, in that spirit, I began to question Evan about the details of pornography's contribution to his nights out on the town.

Evan used cocaine alone, as my most-heavily addicted patients also did. At first I thought Evan sought out pornography as a result of cocaine jacking up his libido. I'd certainly heard *that* story many times before. However, I came to see that I had the order of things reversed. Evan sought out *cocaine* as a result of *pornography* jacking up his libido. This directionality became obvious once the proper questions were asked—Evan had virtually no interest in cocaine unless pornography was available. He rarely used the drug without the filth.

After a while, actual pornography wasn't even required to get the ball rolling. You see, Evan had a singular pattern with smut. He fell smitten with a certain porn actress and followed her *oeuvre* deeply, religiously, for years. With the hours he put in, you can be sure he got to know the essence of her work. In fact, Evan spent so much time intently viewing her films over and over, he could replay extended hardcore sex scenes in his head at will, with impressive graphic detail.

I know the reader's curiosity will be piqued by this obsession, as was mine. Clinicians are not above investigating the artistic objects of their patients' affinities. On many occasions I have perused literature, art, and music in an effort to better acquaint myself with a patient's preferences and influences. Couldn't one argue that, if anything, Evan's *monomaniacal* dedication to one adult film actress rightly *demanded* a serious reconnaissance? How else to even have a shot at understanding this single-minded preoccupation? To experience the films for oneself was the only way to find a potential clue to the mystery. I believe the reader is with me here in principle. Therefore, and in haste, I dutifully found the time and privacy to immerse myself in this most important clinical research.

She had a winning smile, and ably played the part of coquette. Shooting locations favored a tropical clime; a swimming pool often figured early in the exposition. The interior set design was nondescript, and not particularly professional. One quickly discovered that the plotline was contrived and, indeed, unnecessary. The male actors changed in each film, and gave uniformly stiff performances, but our buxom star remained lithe as a ballerina throughout, and stole every show. Overall, the erotic valence was consistently high—at times, the set pieces even seemed to pay homage to early Scandinavian methods. Nevertheless, after careful study, I found nothing in this cinema to distinguish itself from the high-quality mass market. Nor could I wrap my head around Evan's eschewal of the endless erotic novelty of the Internet. To neglect the candy store of this archive for repetitive, memorized choreography from a middle-of-the-pack porn star, however capable her stagecraft, was puzzling. But hey, maybe that's just me.

I wouldn't say my online groundwork was a waste of time, by any means. The films were not aversive, hardly, and led to outcomes expected and unexpected. After long reflection, I concluded that Evan must have a brain whose wiring found this porn star's creative output particularly libidinal and compelling. Why? Who knows? It's the mystery of sexual attraction meeting the mystery of obsession.

The problem for Evan occurred when the films began to play in his head unsolicited. He'd be on his computer at work, focused in on a pressing task, when he would notice his mind had shifted attention *on its own*, and plopped him smack in the middle of a steamy scene he knew by heart. At first, he could wrench himself back to his spreadsheet with moderate mental effort. As time went on though, and Evan continued to stuff the reiterative sex scenes into his memory apparatus, this got harder to do. Film clips of his beloved nymphet—getting it every which way—intruded, unwanted, onto his interior stream of consciousness at inopportune moments, like 3 p.m.

Eventually, a new adaptation emerged. Evan gave up on fighting the images and instead waded into the stream, and let it carry him away. Like anyone else absorbed in a movie, or lost in thought, Evan's "self" disappeared and time stopped temporarily. He became pure disembodied observation—of the carnal circus in his mind's eye—and nothing more. When this hyper-sexual trance state occurred at work, twin irresistible volitions arose: to book a budget hotel room with reliable Internet access, and to procure a supply of cocaine. Both requirements were easily met—one via a simple web search, the other via text to a memorized mobile number. The night was set.

So, getting back to my earlier thesis, the reader now sees why I discounted cocaine as Evan's primary problem. Cocaine was simply a tool to allow, how shall I say, enhanced physiologic responses to extended viewing of his heroine's exploits. Without the smut, there *was* no blow. And without the brain…no problem at all.

I tried many interventions to limit Evan's access to porn, to coke, to cash, to wifi. The rationale was clear and provided a hopeful road map for treatment. Each item proved too laborious to control, however; Evan would always find a workaround. That actually didn't surprise me, although I kept at it nonetheless. Far more difficult was the prospect of trying to control what Evan thought of. That was truly impossible.

SMALL VIGNETTE THREE

Lest the reader feel a rumble to judge, let me clarify that Evan put together many periods of abstinence during our work together. These would not last very long, though; no more than a few months, tops, and often much shorter. I might have prefaced this paragraph with "In my defense," but since I have no illusions my influence meant anything, the amendment would not be fair.

It is also true that throughout the time I thrashed about with Evan's addiction there were significant stretches when he lived in various residential treatment settings. Week upon week of heavy use led to predictable crises, like the risk of job termination, or cardiac arrest, and on several occasions Evan was persuaded to leave town to break the cycle and avoid cataclysm.

Evan never achieved sustained abstinence on my watch, even after discharge from those esteemed New England treatment centers. I had trouble staying ahead of the forces that could upend his fragile sobriety, one of which I just outlined, for any reader still with me, in small vignette two.

Another obstacle to abstinence for Evan, and a universal third-party nemesis for the addiction psychiatrist, was the neighborhood drug dealer. Evan rarely spoke of these shadow players. They were men of few words who operated a text-based delivery service—human kiosks—ideal for our introverted Mr. Evan. He often summoned them as reflex, after the inspiration for porn appeared in his consciousness. Out on the street, the dealer would silently slip Evan the party favor with one hand, while palming the hundreds with the other. No "thank you," no "take it easy."

I ran into a real snag when Evan found a new dealer who was more man than machine. Robert was an acquaintance from AA, someone Evan had formed an arms-length relationship with in the rooms and at the diner afterwards. I considered Robert among the most dangerous of sorts. He frequented AA as a sober poser—not unusual in its own right—but he also used the rooms to troll customers for his cocaine operation. Nice guy.

Based on nothing, I concluded Robert was preying upon Evan; he could see our protagonist's multilayered vulnerabilities and went in for the kill. I cast Robert as an archvillain with formidable powers of psychological manipulation. That made him the exact opposite of me in terms of motive, and effectiveness.

They met often at AA meetings to feign fellowship, and elsewhere to complete the cocaine sales. The exchanges in broad daylight on 96th and Lex struck me as unnecessarily reckless. That was bad enough, but when Evan told me he would sometimes wait at the kitchen table with Robert's grandmother cooking nearby, I feared a sinister bromance had formed.

Accurate or not, the reader can appreciate how these perceptions colored my responses to any reference to Robert. As such, I was particularly challenged the day Evan came in for his session and announced, "I'm in the middle of a drug deal."

"What do you mean?"

"I'm meeting Robert outside in a half hour."

"Robert is coming to meet you in front of the office with cocaine?"

"Yes."

"You've got a hotel room booked for tonight?"

"Yes."

"Why bother coming in to see me then?" I was not pleased.

Evan was looking down now. "We had the appointment set up."

"Yes, that's true…Let's see…What shall we focus on today…?"

Evan didn't like that question.

"You don't need my help completing a drug deal."

"I know!" he fired back immediately. I deserved that.

I toned it down. "If you'd like me to help you not feel like shit tomorrow, and possibly lose your job, I believe I can help."

"Yeah…I know." Resignation.

"Take out your phone. All you have to do is text Robert that you can't make it. We'll find a meeting you can go to instead. Let's call your sponsor."

"I can't…He's on his way already."

"So?? He'll turn around. I'm sure you're not his only customer. He's a big boy; he'll handle it."

"No…I told him I'd meet him."

"Evan, please, this is bullshit. Robert is a drug dealer. You owe him nothing. He will move on to his next customer."

Evan's body began to contract into a ball.

"…He's expecting me…" I was losing him.

"Listen, Evan, let me do this for you. Give me your phone. I'll text Robert and say you've changed your mind.

"I'll call your sponsor," I went on. "In ten minutes we'll have a new plan.

"Think of tomorrow, how much better you'll feel.

"You know you'll dodge a bullet if you don't use tonight."

I had Evan on the ambivalence seesaw now, going back and forth in his head. I pushed a bit more, and he started to reach into his pocket for the phone. *Yes!* He handed it to me.

"What's the number?"

He hesitated. His mouth turned sick. Oh, no. The seesaw began to shift back.

"No, it's okay. I won't meet him. I'll go to a meeting. Let me have the phone back."

"Evan, please, let me shut down the deal. It'll take thirty seconds. Give me his number, and I'll text him. You know you're going to meet him otherwise."

"No, really, it's okay. I'll just go to a meeting."

"Let me call your sponsor right now. I'll ask him to come over and meet you here, then you can go to a meeting with him. What's his number?"

"That's okay. I don't want to call him. Can I have my phone back?"

I tried a couple more times, but he wouldn't budge, insisting instead that he would go to a meeting after the session. He was back to home position. I handed him the phone.

I had one last play, and I had nothing to lose.

"Okay, if you're going to a meeting, then give me your cash. You won't need it. I'll leave it in an envelope with the doorman, and you can pick it up tomorrow."

"I'm not going to meet Robert."

"Oh, yeah? Then you don't need cash."

The challenge led Evan to actually believe for a moment that he had decided to blow off his rendez-vous with Robert. The seesaw started to move again. He stood, pulled out his wallet, and removed a few hundred-dollar bills. *Yes!* I stood to receive, but as he handed them over, the deception could not hold. To see those one hundred dollar banknotes moving through the air towards another man was too much to bear. As far as Evan's brain was concerned, those bills *were* cocaine, and he was already high. He pulled the hundreds back before I could touch them.

"I'm gonna go now. It'll be okay."

Evan left me standing in the middle of the office. I had begged for a good twenty minutes, with nothing to show. It had never been so clear—to meet one's match. There could never be language enough to stop the porn or the coke, at least from me.

I sat down in my chair, and dropped head into hands.

POSTSCRIPT

After he pulled the same stunt a few weeks later—arranging to meet Robert on the corner after a session—Evan and I parted ways. I referred him to a colleague.

CASE NINE

ROMANIAN HOLIDAY

———————•———————

We are generally the better persuaded by the reasons we discover ourselves than by those given to us by others.

—BLAISE PASCAL

AS FAMILY LORE had it, when her marriage to Roman Romanescu produced a son, Mrs. Romanescu was determined he be named after her beloved paternal grandfather, Andrei.

Andrei Tiberius Romanescu was born to a mother devoted to family.

Her husband did not object; he didn't mind "Andrei" at all. But Roman was the kind of man who never passed up the chance for quid pro quo. He moaned that the allowance of "Andrei" was a great concession on his part and, as compensation, asked for carte blanche on the selection of the *middle* name for the child, paltry consolation though it was. Mrs. R. fell for his ruse hook, line, and sinker and consented, secretly believing she got the better end of the deal. That's the best con—when the mark feels they've conned the con man.

Roman pitched his wife some BS about how Tiberius would be a clever play on "Roman" roots, a wry but nonsensical association since the Romanescu lineage was about as pure Eastern European as they come. The actual motive for "Tiberius" was far more pedestrian—Roman was a big fan of Star Trek—especially the character of James T. Kirk. No matter, Mrs. R. was diverted by the glamour of a Roman pedigree and forever looked upon Tiberius with admiration. And so this episode illustrated two fixed features of Mrs. R.'s character: devotion and credulity.

───────────●───────────

Mrs. Romanescu herself made the initial call to me on Andrei's behalf. She had spoken to a few psychiatrists before obtaining my number. They each demurred on the case after hearing her brief description of Andrei's situation. Mrs. R. thought she had interviewed these psychiatrists as potential clinicians for Andrei, but the reality was that the psychiatrists had evaluated *her*, surrogate though she was, and she had horribly botched every audition.

"Doctor, my son Andrei has a terrible addiction to heroin. He's been to rehab six times. We've spent $250,000 on treatment for him over the past ten years. He's never worked a day in his life. Doctor, something is seriously wrong with Andrei. We give him a wonderful life. He has no interest in anything, just the drugs. There must be a reason. No one has figured it out. What can you do to help us?"

"Mrs. Romanescu, I'm so sorry you and your family have gone through this. You've certainly made an extraordinary effort to help your son. The only thing I can do is an evaluation to see if anything has been overlooked, but I doubt it."

Sold! She accepted the lukewarm offer on the spot, no questions asked, and I felt a faint nausea brew within. I thought of the string of colleagues who had passed up the same opportunity, chuckling somewhere.

———————•———————

Mrs. Romanescu brought Andrei to the first visit and parked herself in the waiting room. She would do that for every visit. Andrei was not allowed to travel anywhere by himself as a condition of living at home. Travel would be difficult in any case as Andrei was not permitted to hold any money and had none of his own. Mrs. R. handed me an envelope and explained, "I filled out your registration form for Andrei."

"Thank you." I motioned for the patient to enter the inner office.

As we settled into our chairs, I said, "Let me look at the form before we start."

If based only on the bold cursive with which Mrs. R. had written his name on my registration form, I might have thought Andrei Tiberius Romanescu was actually descended from Romanian aristocracy. But in America it's the address that counts—and reveals more about family history than any name ever could. And so my eye, perked by the patrician calligraphy, naturally fell to the next line of the form with a certain expectation—where *do* the ex-pat descendants of Romanian gentry live in the Tri-State area?

You can imagine my surprise when I discovered the Romanescu's address to be within the hamlet of my own childhood—Richmond Hill, Queens.

There's much one can say about multicultural, working class Queens—I recently read two hundred languages were spoken there—but one fact is ironclad: it is *not* the obvious choice for the emigration of elites from *any* nation-state, save those seeking to escape serious scandal or who need some other reason for witness-protection obscurity.

Specifically, they lived on Park Lane South, the winding boulevard that hugs the boundary of Forest Park, that improbable 538 acres of splendid woodland. This put the Romanescus on the ostensible gold coast of Richmond Hill, with the distinct chance that at least one of their windows looked out onto a fine urban green space. For most of the other properties in Richmond Hill that were not on Park Lane South, windows tended to look out onto a modest, close-set neighbor in a struggle of some sort.

Given the address, the next logical question was how the Romanescus came to Manhattan to explore treatment for their son. Manhattan addiction services were typically set at an absurdly high, fixed price point—one that discouraged shrewd Richmond Hill shoppers accustomed to browbeating vendors into bargain-basement submission. That turned out to be self-explanatory—the family business logo was embossed on the envelope. "Romanescu Waste Management" opened all kinds of doors, and in Queens was as close to a limitless checkbook a family could have—and far more informative than any address even.

I looked up from the form and took note that Andrei was muscular, and I wondered whether he had spent time in a penitentiary weight room given the risks of his preferred activities. He would later acknowledge arrests for petty burglary, but Andrei's physique was not a product of extended incarceration. I began the formal consultation with a variant of my standard opening, reserved for circumstances such as these.

"As you know, your mother arranged this consultation. What's your understanding of why we're meeting?"

"Mom said you had something to offer."

Ah, already a misunderstanding, right out of the gate. Inflated expectations, no doubt dangled by Mrs. R. to coax her son to Manhattan.

"What's the issue?"

"Can't stop doing heroin."

Andrei clarified a few things off the bat. He was sitting with me forty-six days clean, which sounded pretty respectable to me, but then again he added that he'd just been in rehab for forty-five of the forty-six. And it was more like fifteen stints in addiction treatment facilities if you counted detox, wilderness, and sober living in addition to rehab. And that didn't include the encyclopedia that, if it existed, would contain the outpatient records. It looked as though Andrei hadn't been able to put together even two weeks clean outside of a controlled environment. The part about not working a day in his life was accurate.

"How did it all start?"

Now thirty years old, Andrei began to explore the basics of street pharmacology in adolescence, in typical Richmond Hill High School fashion, which is to say with cheap beer, cheap weed, and fast friends, deep in a verdant glen of Forest Park. That would have been fine by itself, and shared by half of the RHHS student body, but Andrei grew bored of mild euphorics and found a clique that, like him, fancied stronger tonics. And so cocaine, psychedelics, and heroin joined the party. Andrei took to heroin quickly. Heroin turned something on in Andrei's brain that never quite turned off.

For the past ten-plus years Andrei's life had simplified down to a few behaviors: getting heroin, using heroin, and managing the inevitable consequences therein. Arguably, a common garden snail expresses a wider behavioral repertoire. At this level of exposure, the human brain becomes accustomed to a bathwater of heroin, and finds a way to keep it so. Andrei himself told me that the urge to use was never far away and mostly impossible to resist. The best he could do was to briefly forget his circumstances, like a person recently bereaved, until something cued a memory for the yearned object.

It wouldn't take long for that something to occur. One of Andrei's most powerful triggers for heroin was women, and he appeared to have an endless supply of female contacts eager to use with him and then have sex. Texts that enticed were never too far in the future, it seemed. A fine double trouble.

After the failed investment of two hundred fifty large to beat back heroin, Andrei was ready to get to the bottom of things. He had some ideas. Andrei was an only child and wondered if he had grown up spoiled. There *was* a faint streak of self-centeredness within his decision-making. Also, he was not a good student—something about not seeing the board clearly. That could be relevant to the undeveloped work history.

These were important observations, I commented, certainly worth a deep excavation, but I had another thought in addition. It was hard to believe, but after all those years of treatment Andrei had never been given a trial of the opioid blocker naltrexone. This simple medicine blocks any opioid drug from activating its receptor, thereby preventing the high. He seemed the poster child for the molecule.

Andrei knew all about naltrexone. He wasn't interested. He wanted to work on his issues, and he was getting a little testy with my soliloquy on the power of receptor blockade to prevent re-addiction, protect against accidental overdose, and maybe speed up receptor re-regulation. Just then Andrei mentioned that his rehab had referred him to an outpatient facility for aftercare, and the intake was scheduled for next week. I took that to signal he was done with me for today, and maybe forever, especially if the outpatient facility turned out to be more sympathetic to an exploration of his "issues," rather than to annoying blocker medications.

"Why don't you complete your assessment with the outpatient program then call me back for a follow-up?"

Andrei agreed.

I gave it a 25 percent chance.

———————•———————

Two months later Mrs. R. called to arrange the follow-up. Andrei had rejected the outpatient program, and that left him sitting at home with idle hands. Not good. The texts from women continued to roll in during this period of unstructured home confinement, and we know what that meant. It made me wonder why Mr. and Mrs. Romanescu didn't confiscate Andrei's phone. I suppose that might be considered a criminal level of deprivation these days.

Andrei had used heroin fifteen times over this interval. His parents pressured him to accept a local outpatient program three nights a week. He was back to start therapy with me to understand why he became an addict. I knew that this was Mrs. Romanescu's wish, to get at the causes of the devastation, but I couldn't tell whether Andrei truly shared this agenda or was giving me lip service. When he announced his willingness to take naltrexone in pill form (it also comes in a long-acting injection form), I gave him the benefit of the doubt.

We walked together to the waiting room and I told Mrs. R. that Andrei and I would begin regular, weekly sessions. I explained the use of naltrexone, and that Andrei had a prescription and should start today. Mrs. R. was very happy to hear this news. She thanked me profusely and began to rub Andrei's back with parental tenderness. He looked down as she stroked, timid. As they left I heard her repeat, "Very good, Andrei, very good…"

The first two therapy sessions were encouraging. Andrei was blocked on naltrexone and abstinent from heroin. He was attending the outpatient program. I detected a glimmer of curiosity from Andrei—curiosity about how addiction altered his mind. This was a very good sign; without curiosity, therapy is often just a technical exercise, like building an IKEA bookcase.

Andrei had started an online class in basic mathematics, part of an initiative to develop marketable skills, and immediately became frustrated with a problem set. The naltrexone blockade prevented reflexive heroin use and allowed Andrei a pause to observe his reactions. As uncomfortable as this was, Andrei could see clearly that the math challenge led to a strong desire to drop the class and a stronger desire to use heroin. From this he began to construct a useful model of how negative emotions evoked cravings for heroin and how his lifelong need for instant gratification sealed his fate. We were off to the races.

Between Andrei's first and second sessions, I had an awkward exchange with Mrs. R. She had developed a bit of a habit herself—to call and leave messages detailing Andrei's actions and state of mind. After the first of Andrei's therapy sessions, she left a message asking me to return her call. She picked up when I called back.

"Doctor, Andrei is responding to the therapy. He is taking his medicine and attending his classes. He seems happier and is helping around the house. I want to thank you."

"That's great. He's learning some important things about addiction."

"One thing I noticed, doctor, is that your fee went up."

"Oh, I'm sorry, I thought we went over that in the initial phone call. I started out seeing Andrei as a medication case. That session is thirty minutes at the lower fee. When we switched to the therapy sessions, I put him into the forty-five minute therapy slot at the higher fee."

"I see. But doctor, Andrei has been through a lot of treatment. We've spent $250,000. And Andrei really likes working with you. Doctor, please, can you keep seeing him for the lower fee?"

It seemed a reasonable request. Maybe waste management wasn't limitless after all. Or maybe everything was a negotiation for the Romanescus. It didn't matter. I wasn't going to treat this like a carpet salesman.

"Of course. I understand. We'll keep it at the lower fee."

———•———

The third session started to show some cracks. Andrei had used over the past weekend. A co-patient at the outpatient program told him if he stopped naltrexone, by the next day he could get high. The proposition was enough to fuel a strong urge. When that cute girl in his process group offered another proposition, the deal was done. He found his mother's wallet, then the car keys, then was gone. The girl had a soft spot for speedballs, heroin plus cocaine, and Andrei the gentleman extended his strong arm and ably escorted her all evening.

I brought Mrs. R. into the office to join us.

"This is a setback, no question, and it shows the limits of naltrexone in pill form. Much more powerful is the naltrexone injection, known as Vivitrol. This is a shot into the muscle of the buttock that leeches out the blocker over three to four weeks, so there's no getting high for that time period, no matter what triggers come along."

Andrei looked dejected. "Vivitrol won't make a difference. I'll just use something else…coke, crack, meth…"

That was almost certainly true, but still, did that warrant rejecting Vivitrol? When I consider the insulation needs of my house, I see that there will be some heat loss from the chimney that I cannot prevent, but do I then abandon *all* insulation in response?

Mrs. R. chimed in, "Andrei, you should listen to what the doctor is saying."

A tepid endorsement to be sure. I had hoped for something more forceful from Mrs. R., something with the weight of a quarter-million dollars behind it. After all, she was willing to use the figure with me.

Andrei sat silent. His body appeared bolted to the floor.

I decided not to waste my insulation metaphor on the Romanescus. There would be no Vivitrol; I had to accept that. But Andrei's rejection of injectable naltrexone was a dire sign. Without reliable blockade from heroin assured, and in light of the titillating possibilities at the outpatient program, Andrei was not going to make it very far. From the get-go I thought this case would end with an inpatient referral sooner or later, given the history. Now was the time to start prepping the family. I had a specific treatment in mind.

"I hate to be alarmist about it, but I think we should seriously consider another inpatient treatment for Andrei. I don't know if he can stay clean under the current conditions. Maybe something long-term, much longer than thirty days."

An excited Mrs. R. jumped in, "Doctor, Andrei has seen it all. It doesn't make a difference. The rehabs are all the same. He relapses immediately. We've been through this so many times." Then came the inevitable, "Doctor, we cannot afford another $50,000 vacation."

"I agree Andrei has seen expensive, traditional inpatient treatment over and over. And the results are not great. But there's another kind of treatment that costs far less than a 30-day rehab and provides months of inpatient care, sometimes up to a year. It's called a therapeutic community, and it doesn't get as much attention as it should.

"The model is very different—it's not about rehabilitation, it's about *habilitation*—the idea that some patients need to learn pro-social behaviors from scratch, from the basics. Values of self-help and mutual-help are taught in real time within the therapeutic community. In fact, living and contributing to the community *is* the treatment. Patients develop skills and a sense of pride rotating through different jobs that keep the community functioning. The patients run all elements of the community, with staff support and oversight. Patients receive coaching on things like conflict resolution, how to take criticism, how to prepare for a job interview, and many other practical skills.

"Given Andrei's extensive history of addiction and absence of work experience, I think he would benefit from a long program that teaches its members to contribute and function productively in a community. I don't think he's ever done that."

I finished my pitch and looked at son and mother.

"I don't want to go away again. Definitely not for a year."

Mrs. R. showed a touch of daylight, "Doctor, maybe you could send me some information on this program. How much does it cost?"

OK, that wasn't too bad for the first round. This was a project that would take multiple conversations.

"Of course, I'll get you the name of a program. Why don't we put Andrei back on the naltrexone pill for now?"

Therapeutic communities are in fact less often considered in addiction treatment, and it had been a long time since I researched one for a patient. I called on an old colleague, an expert in TCs, and asked for a recommendation for a patient like Andrei. He suggested an outfit off the grid in New Mexico, and after looking at their website I passed the info to Mrs. R., then waited for her to let the concept percolate.

But events in the Romanescu case unfolded faster than I expected. On the morning of the scheduled fourth session, exactly a week after the conspicuous third session, Mrs. R. called to cancel. I phoned her back and learned Andrei had had a bad relapse. He went AWOL for 36 hours, presumably with the same girl from outpatient. The extended binge didn't go well for him. I suspected he might have hit the cocaine too hard because Mrs. R. described a clear paranoid reaction. She found Andrei cowering behind the front bushes of the house, babbling about his need to keep a low profile from the police. The fact that he was naked lent support to my theory.

The TC in New Mexico was looking prescient, but Mrs. R. wasn't there yet. Andrei cleared the cocaine, and the paranoid psychosis resolved. The relapse made no dent in his resistance to go inpatient. He cast the episode as a one-off anomaly, a case of tainted cocaine that would not happen again, and swore off the girl. Without a willing partner, and facing the prospect of another five-figure price tag, albeit low five-figure, Mrs. R. caved on the TC, and we went back to poor, beleaguered oral naltrexone.

Everyone ought to be given time to accept the reality of their condition. I scheduled the Romanescus for the same slot next week.

———————•———————

The day came and with it another call in the morning from Mrs. R. to cancel. Andrei had relapsed once more. There was something about this one though; Mrs. R. had already called the TC and was arranging the admission.

"What happened?"

"Doctor, you were right. Andrei must go away. He cannot stay in our house."

"Mrs. Romanescu, did something happen in the house?"

"Doctor, I have a safe in the basement for years, because of all the things that Andrei has stolen. I keep everything in there now—cash, checkbooks, jewelry, anything of value. Last week I went downstairs to put some cash in. Later that day Andrei disappeared with the car. I had a funny feeling and went to check the safe. Doctor, all the money was gone. I didn't know how he did it. The combination is not written down anywhere, and he wasn't in the basement when I opened it.

"When Andrei finally got home high, I got it out of him. Doctor, do you know what he did? He hid behind the washing machine for hours waiting for me to come down. He found the perfect spot to see me open the safe. He memorized the combination. Doctor, he sat behind the washing machine for hours quiet as a mouse."

That was it for Mrs. Romanescu.

"Andrei is very sick doctor; he is going to New Mexico."

"I'm sorry, Mrs. Romanescu. But I think you're making the right decision."

———————•———————

Over the next few months Mrs. Romanescu left me a series of voicemail messages. Initially a bit cautious, her messages grew more joyous and grateful over time as she described Andrei's radical, positive transformation at the TC. Numerous letters from Andrei, and a weekly live phone call with him, convinced the Romanescus that their son might have licked his addiction. I responded to her first call and was, of course, supportive. Nevertheless, despite my own recommendation of the TC, given the depth of Andrei's addiction I wasn't about to take any credit just yet. I didn't respond to Mrs. R.'s messages past the first one, although I listened to them. She was so proud of her son. I hoped she was right, but I remained guarded.

Mrs. Romanescu possibly interpreted my silence as skepticism, or maybe my ambivalence came through plainly in the call we had. I say this because a few months after he went away, Mrs. R. sent me a photocopy of a letter she had received from Andrei. Handwritten by him, the unedited text went as follows:

Dear, Mom, & Dad.

Hello From Las Cruces, never thought I would say that. I want to thank you for this opportunity to trully find myself. This place is very good. I am living in a community of 80-100 men & women that help each other and the community every day. I have spent many years on heroin as you know and In the dark. Being around people is the best thing for me. We group every day along with work around the ranch. I did some landscaping and helped the kitchen.

So far I have been doing good. today is 2 weeks clean and I actually see my faults in others, myself and thru the interactions with others. There are people here that I can tell anything. All the times I was angry it was just my own frustration when I thought the world was out to get me, it cause I don't know how to communicate when I am insecure, its cause I do no estemable acts. So much of what you and Dad have told me growing up. All of these little philosophys and ways to look at life. This place is beautiful. How are you? How is dad? How is the weather? its wierd for the first time in my life Im not looking to run or get over. I pray every night and every morning when I get up. I pray to stay humble and learn about myself so I leave here with a set of tools I can face the world with and fix my problems head on. Thank you and Dr. Mierlak as well.

Love,
Andrei

Hey, maybe she *was* right.
Finally, we might have a happy ending!

POSTSCRIPT

Exactly eight months after cracking the safe, Andrei was back in my office. Mrs. Romanescu set up the visit. She called a week before Andrei's discharge, and with the return to Richmond Hill imminent, she hoped he and I could resume our therapy together. As was her habit, Mrs. Romanescu stayed in the waiting room while Andrei and I met.

He was deeply tanned. The months of outdoor work in the desert had pumped him up, and Andrei now looked like a bronzed bodybuilder. He seemed more relaxed than I remembered, and he took his usual spot on the couch with a friendly smile.

"Welcome back. How was the experience?"

"You spoke to my mother?"

"A bit. She left messages with updates on your progress. Sent me a copy of the letter you wrote home after two weeks there."

"Yeah. The place was interesting. I'm done with drugs. That I know for sure."

"That's great. It sounds like the program really helped you."

"How much do you know about that program?"

"I've never referred anyone to that specific program, but I know a fair amount about TCs. I worked in one earlier in my career. I thought it would be a good fit for you given all the rehabs you tried. I called my old supervisor for a recommendation. He suggested the Las Cruces program."

Andrei stopped smiling.

"Have you ever visited that program?"

"No, I haven't. As I said, I asked an old teacher for the recommendation."

"You sent me to a place you never saw. For eight months. You think that's right? You think that's the right thing to do to a person? To send them away for eight months to a place you never laid eyes on, never saw for yourself?"

"What happened there? I thought you found the experience helpful."

"I'm done with drugs. I'll give the place that. But it was a hellhole. Filled with ex-cons looking to avoid jail. Half the time I was afraid for my life. Learned more about getting over than I ever knew. Living conditions were horrible. Woke up covered in bites the first week. Roommate and I took our beds out and burned them. Worked us to the bone—day, night, brutal heat, whatever. No let-up. Part of the learning experience they said. You're free to go if you want, they'd say; but we were in the middle of nowhere in the desert."

"Oh my God. I'm sorry to hear this. I had no idea."

"Yeah, I know you didn't. Because you never visited the place. You sent a patient you were supposed to help to a place you never looked at. Mr. Substance Abuse Expert. You just made a phone call and dumped me into a fucking meat grinder for eight months."

This was not going well. Andrei turned menacing.

"I've been thinking about this visit for a while now. I've been thinking about how much I got hurt in Las

Cruces and how it was your fault. Because you didn't give a fuck about doing the work to research this place. Made a phone call and charged my mother's AMEX. Got me out of your hair for eight months. I've been thinking you're a shit doctor who fucked up with the wrong person, and you need to be taught a lesson so you won't do this to another patient."

I was riveted, not in a good way.

"I've been thinking I should lay a beating on you right now that would hurt you like you hurt me. One that you won't ever forget. You won't ever make the same mistake with another patient. I'll walk away sure of *that*."

I've always looked at my childhood and adolescence in Queens, for all of its limitations, as giving me the street smarts to successfully navigate challenging circumstances. The first significant exception to this construct was my 1985 visit to Christiana, the anarchist enclave in Copenhagen, where I became aware of a new kind of fear within the lawlessness of that place. Now, with just a few choice sentences, Andrei kicked up that Christiana feeling again.

"But because my mother is in the waiting room, I will not beat the shit out of you. I can see by looking at you my message has gotten through. Don't ever fuck with someone's life and send them to a shithole you don't know. Next time you might not be so lucky."

Andrei sat back, and after a few seconds I realized he was finished with his piece. He stared at me with icy, unblinking eyes set within an expressionless face, in total command of the moment. He waited for my response.

For a minute there, for the first time in my career, I expected a patient to assault me in my own office. And I accepted that the assault would be violent, overwhelming, and indefensible. Just as quick, Andrei made the expectation evaporate, and the paralysis of the Christiana effect lifted. I was able to think again, and more importantly, I was able to remember I came from Queens, too.

"I take your point, Andrei. I won't do that again."

He still hadn't blinked.

"I have a thought. Why don't we go to the waiting room and I'll tell your mother that you don't need to see me for therapy."

"That would be a good idea, doctor." He finally blinked.

"I agree. Let's go right now."

If Mrs. Romanescu was surprised by the session ending early, she didn't show it. She was reading the paper when I opened the door to the waiting room; and when she looked up and made eye contact with me, she let out a big smile. Andrei walked past me and stood beside his mother, crossed his arms, and let out his own big smile. You could see the family resemblance in the mouth. I spoke to Mrs. R.

"It's so nice to see Andrei healthy. He's doing great. The program really did a good job for him. In fact, since he's not on medicine, he doesn't need to see me."

"Really, doctor? But what about the therapy?"

"Andrei and I agree that's not needed at the moment. He learned a lot of skills in New Mexico. If things change, you can always call me back; but Andrei and I are confident he doesn't need to see me right now."

Mrs. R. looked up at her son. "Andrei, you're okay with not seeing Dr. Mierlak?"

"The doc knows what he's talking about."

She stood up. "Andrei is doing so well. We have our son back thanks to you, doctor. We will follow your advice. Thank you so much."

Mrs. Romanescu reached out and took my right hand into both of hers and shook it with deep gratitude. When she finished, Andrei grabbed the same hand and squeezed painfully hard, then gave me a wink.

I opened and held the office outer door for them, and, after they left, I counted to three and threw the lock.

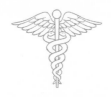

I NOW PRONOUNCE YOU DEAD

———————•———————

In the year before I started the specialized training to become a psychiatrist, long before I knew anything about addiction psychiatry, I had the rare privilege to work as an intern across several medical settings. The experience left a lasting impression.

For most of that year I wore a hideous white blazer over cheap button-down shirts and ties. The short white coat is the standard uniform for interns. It is cut from fabric that could not have originated with any plant or animal species native to our planet.

Initially, I recoiled at the garment as a fashion grotesquerie. It was only later I realized the importance to protect oneself from stain.

THE MODERN GAME of Medicine is played at its highest levels and with the highest stakes inside a thing called the teaching hospital. In Manhattan, New York Hospital was just such a place, and on its campus the imposing Baker Tower housed the inpatient units. Entire floors were dedicated to the treatment of Medicine patients, whose diseases included everything that wasn't covered by the surgery, pediatrics, neurology, or obstetrics services. A single Medicine floor was large enough to support multiple clinical teams, each chronically overworked by the burden of caring for their portion of some seriously diseased real estate.

On certain floors, including Baker 16, where I had the privilege to serve, there was a partitioned area at one end that contained a few oversized private rooms, much like the first-class section of a commercial airliner. This was where the shah of Iran, Richard Nixon, Andy Warhol, and other notables with special privacy needs got treated. You could also get treated there if you donated substantial sums of money to the hospital, or if you were rich and got sick and might later become someone who donated substantial sums of money.

To be fair, ordinary citizens were sometimes placed in these special rooms as well, if the VIPs happened to be out of town. After a couple weeks of internship, the patients in the partitioned wing held no allure. Disease looks and smells exactly the same in every room on Baker 16, I can assure you, regardless of the fame or net worth of the occupant. And disease is the only reason anyone comes to Baker 16.

All of which segues nicely to the final night in the life of the unfortunate Mr. A.D. Lombardi, inpatient at New York Hospital, Baker 16 Medicine service.

Insider tip: in Medicine, when they use the adjective "unfortunate" in the identifying information, the patient has a disease that is very, very bad. For example, if the top line of a summary reads, "Mr. A.D. Lombardi is an unfortunate fifty-three-year-old, married, Caucasian male with congestive heart failure admitted to Baker 16," you can be sure Mr. Lombardi has a very, very bad case of congestive heart failure and will likely die from it. He's unfortunate—he's had some very bad luck.

In contrast to the unfortunate A.D. Lombardi, the final night of his life was, for me, just another unsavory night on call as an intern on the Baker 16 Medicine service.

As 6 p.m. approached on the day whose night would be A.D. Lombardi's last, my fellow interns were getting ready to punch out. They had busted their asses on patient care all day, and they were itching to sign out their caseloads and beat it. While the pace of scheduled tasks would slow overnight, remember this was a floor full of very sick people, with active disease processes that didn't abide a 7-to-6 workday. Patients crashed in the wee hours all the time. Tending to one sick patient who de-tuned could keep you busy until dawn.

They took turns handing me printouts of their cases. I scribbled notes beside the patients who had tests to follow up on, or who needed a specific intervention that night, or who were teetering and needed someone to keep an eye on them. It was all very serious stuff, and every detail would have to be attended to.

During the staccato rundown of the sign-out, the instructions for Lombardi initially didn't faze me because they were not complicated.

"Lombardi's got end-stage CHF and needs to be diuresed. He's got terrible access, so you'll have to push the Lasix. He gets a shot q four."

Translation: Mr. Lombardi had advanced conges-tive heart failure and was near the point where Medicine's medicines neared the end of their abil-ity to keep him alive. His heart was failing as a pump—it couldn't push enough blood through his kidneys to make appropriate amounts of urine. As a result, his body accumulated fluid. To try to compensate, we would give him Lasix, a drug that increased the production of urine (diuresis). Mr. Lombardi's veins were too compromised to hold a fixed IV, so each dose of Lasix would be given by hand by the intern, "pushed" via injection from a single-use hypodermic needle into whatever vein could be located. Every four hours.

Then came the kicker.
"He's gonna die tonight. Don't worry, he's DNR."

Translation: Mr. Lombardi was expected to die tonight. He carried the somber status "Do Not Resuscitate," which meant he or his official health designate had requested that heroic resuscitation measures not be initiated if his heart stopped beating. I did not have to worry tonight since I would not have to initiate said heroic measures to resuscitate him when his heart finally gave out from end-stage congestive heart failure.

―――――――――●―――――――――

When you've got a million things to do in a set amount of time, no single thing stands out. You just work down your list and hope no curveball, like a spike of fever or a bloody vomitus, clogs up your progress. And so it was for me that night on call. I worked my list, bundling tasks to improve efficiency, and hoped a lull would occur eventually to allow a catnap.

Lombardi's first shot of Lasix was scheduled for 10 p.m. I was still in pretty good shape—the night was young, no one had crashed, and I found the time to order and completely consume a burger and fries. At 10:05, I gathered the supplies to inject Lombardi with the medicine that would help his kidneys make urine.

He was in one of the VIP rooms of Baker 16's partitioned area. As I headed over, I wondered if his family had some clout. The question inspired a second or two of reflection but led to no associations, so was discarded. Immediately another thought arose. I found myself irritated by the discovery that the VIP section, far from the nurse's station, was a pain in the ass to walk to when on call.

Oddly enough, upon entering Lombardi's room, it was the light I noticed first. The overhead fluorescent bulbs seemed turned up too high, and emitted a bright, nauseating light bath that filled the room. I suppose the point was to provide more illumination to help people like me perform procedures or conduct examinations, but the quality of the glow would make any person look more sickly than they already were. And Lombardi looked plenty sick irrespective of light source.

The only soul in the chamber, he lay on a hospital bed asleep on his back, with a standard-issue white sheet pulled up to half-chest. It's hard to tell a person's height when he lies in a hospital bed, so I cannot comment on that. However, I could see that his hair remained enviously brown for a middle-aged man, and that would turn out to be the extent of Lombardi's normal features. Even before I pulled the sheet down to expose his arms, I knew something was terribly wrong with Mr. Lombardi.

The man retained so much fluid that his entire body had swelled. It was as though someone attached him to an air hose at a gas station and walked away. He was overfilled to the point that he appeared a human-sized zeppelin. The expected topography of a body, the creases and bumps and lines, had disappeared. I understood why no IV could be placed—there was no vein near the surface of his skin. They were all submerged to various depths beneath a layer of edema fluid that by rights should have been pissed away awhile ago, if he had a heart that could pump a damn. His chest moved or I might've thought him dead already.

Where was the family if this was A.D. Lombardi's last night? Why no vigil? He certainly deserved one, didn't he? I scanned his spacious quarters; the room was a perfect hybrid of hospital and hotel. Lombardi's side had all the functional plastic and metal hardware common to every other patient room on Baker 16. His sitting area, however, a generous bump-out that tripled the square footage, was decorated with an eye to evoke the lobby of the Carlyle. Furnished with finely uphol-stered wing chairs and Chesterfield, it was typically occupied by a toney entourage that oozed of money and power.

As I looked at Lombardi and thought about it further, maybe it was better no one was here. I had a job to do, and it was going to be one heck of a technical challenge. In order to get Lasix into his bloodstream, I would have to harpoon one of Lombardi's invisible veins with my syringe.

———————•———————

I was skeptical of tying a tourniquet on his upper arm, a technique that normally compressed the underlying vein and caused blood to back up and bulge the vessel. Lombardi's arms were so swollen, it would be as if I placed a strap around a cylinder of foam rubber and tightened, the tension creating a circular indentation that cut a deep groove, of dubious function. Even if the hidden vein could be compressed and enlarged by the maneuver, it would still be a blind stab to try to spear it.

I fastened the tourniquet nonetheless, figuring my odds for success would be zero without it, so why not try? The skin of his antecubital fossa (pit of the elbow— the standard spot for venipuncture) went taut as a drum—stretched into a smooth, thin, and translucent membrane that strained against the volume within. Looking down at the area, the neophyte might fear to puncture it lest clear fluid shoot out.

To penetrate Lombardi's vein wall and deliver the 5 cc Lasix payload, I chose the more muscular 20-gauge needle for the job, foolishly reasoning a larger bore would make it easier to push liquid medicine through. This would be seen later as pure fantasy physics.

The left antecubital fossa was swabbed with an isopropyl alcohol pad. I homed in on my mark, a spot on the skin somewhere left of center, with the hypodermic held in an underhand grip—the way you'd hold a prison shiv, albeit with more tenderness. The angle of approach was surprisingly shallow, certainly sub-30 degrees, and the forward motion deliberate and steady.

The 20-gauge stainless steel needle had a deviously sharp beveled tip. It popped Lombardi's bubble-skin effortlessly and, meeting no resistance, was half an inch down before I jammed on the brakes. I looked over at Lombardi's face. No reaction. After a slight readjustment to my grip, I began a careful advance of the needle forward and down, while simultaneously pulling back a touch on the syringe's plunger with my other hand. This created a small negative pressure within the chamber of the syringe. When the needle's tip pierced the vein, blood would rush in and backfill the syringe—visual evidence that I had entered the bloodstream. Then a quick, second adjustment to the grip and I could smoothly depress the plunger, confident that the injection would enter the interior of the circulatory system. That, anyway, was the theory, and the hope.

The needle advanced, and advanced, and advanced, but no blood returned. I pushed it slow, but Jesus, where was the vessel? Then, KA-CLUNK, I hit and scraped an iceberg: *BONE*. Shit. I hit bone. The collision of super-sharp steel with live bone—such a rookie blunder—mortified me, and caused a slight, reflexive, backwards yank on the needle. That *had* to be an exquisite spasm of pain. Again I looked over to Lombardi's face, and again I saw no hint of a flinch. The man could not have had much left in the world of the living to not feel that.

Humbled, grateful for no witnesses, and with the needle still in his arm, I resumed my fishing expedition—this time employing short stabs in an effort to hook Lombardi's pesky vein. Back and forth I lunged, aware that I risked nicking bone, tendon, or nerve, but secure in the knowledge it would not register for unfortunate Lombardi.

After a few such attempts, I realized I was just hacking away pointlessly; the vein could not be breached. I looked down, to a bag that hung below the mattress. Lombardi had a hose attached to his penis, the other end of which terminated in the bag. Any urine Lombardi voided would travel that hose and collect in the bag. It was empty. I looked back to my hands that held the hypodermic shoved into Lombardi's bloated arm. How much further should I desecrate his body in the service of injecting medicine into his bloodstream? Medicine that was likely to do nothing.

Fuck it. I released the negative pressure on the syringe, gripped the thing firmly, and squeezed the entire bolus into some random space within Lombardi's elbow. So he got his Lasix after all. Box checked. I cleaned up and left the room.

After that misadventure, I went back to my list, which hadn't gotten any shorter during my time in Lombardi's room. There were IVs to place, blood cultures to draw, tests to follow up on...

Before I knew it, it was 2 a.m., time for Lombardi's next shot. Fatigue had set in; there had been no break in the workflow, and I was getting punchy. I gathered the supplies and headed back down the hall to his room.

Lombardi hadn't moved. He was still breathing. I went around the bed and checked the bag for urine. It was still empty. The nurses record vital signs and various other metrics of the live human body on a clipboard kept at the bedside. I picked it up and saw that Lombardi hadn't made any urine for the past two shifts—sixteen hours.

This now struck me as imbecilic. Lombardi was in renal failure—his kidneys were shut down and could not make urine. And, he was in a coma, impervious to deep pain. The remainder of Lombardi's life was a matter of hours. The Lasix exercise was utterly useless. Why was it still on the books? Was it a remnant of earlier interventions for CHF, overlooked as the others were systematically pulled back? Or did the family request it—a relatively benign Hail Mary pass that would allow them to feel they hadn't given up on him? And where the hell *was* the family? Surely they were told he was on the brink? Not one person here to hold his hand, to tell him he was loved and would be missed, just in case some tendril of auditory awareness endured? Who *were* these people? What kind of family abandons kin on the cusp of death?

I didn't know why Lombardi was alone. I could tell nothing of his life at this moment. The richness of his story—when he soared, or failed, what he held dear—none of it was available to me. He was a bloated body, naked and beached upon a hospital bed, in a room sickly lit, at the end of a Medicine ward. But there *was* a story to Lombardi even if I didn't know it, and he deserved a witness to honor it as his end approached.

We don't always get what we deserve. Lombardi would not have his witness. But, he would also not have any further disturbance to his body. I turned and left the room, and returned the vial of Lasix and other supplies to where they belonged.

The nurse came to me at 4 a.m. I was in the station, bleary-eyed now, trying my best to cross-reference test results from the computer screen with my scribbled list. Lombardi had died. She found him dead on her rounds.

I suppose it makes sense that experts who specialize in caring for the living should be called on to certify when life has ended. It's an event of great importance to families, and to the individual involved, of course, although for very different reasons. To verify death is one of the solemn duties of physicians. Personally, I don't see why nurses can't attest to death when it occurs in the hospital—they're certainly qualified, and often have a keener sense of what has been lost when a patient dies. I guess it's another thing we have to chalk up to tradition. A very old tradition at that.

Few procedures of modern Medicine can claim a through line back to antiquity. The ritual of pronouncing a patient dead is just such an example, and it has changed little with the passage of millennia. Indeed, not only would Babylonian physicians recognize the modern version, they would be quite competent at administering the protocol.

I consider myself fortunate to have pronounced dead only a couple of patients, far fewer than I've seen die first-hand. Most of the time another doctor had primary responsibility. Tonight, though, it was just me on Baker 16, and it was my duty to pronounce Lombardi—this was not the kind of thing an intern woke the second-year resident for—even if Lombardi was to be my first ever.

———•———

Entering Lombardi's room for the third time, I needed no special instruments to complete the task that now found itself at the top of my list. Everything required was already part of my permanent tool kit: stethoscope, penlight, and my own eyes, ears, and fingers. The nurse had turned the overhead lights off; only the panel above the headboard illuminated the room. It too cast that fluorescent hue, but at least the wattage had come down considerably. She had done another thing also; she had pulled the white sheet up over Lombardi's head so that his entire body lay underneath, concealed from view— the universal sign that the irregular mound on the bed was a corpse.

Why does the image of a corpse evoke fear? The very word seen in print can be enough to stir disquiet. Try it out, now:

CORPSE.

Images of death reach down to the deepest visceral instincts. And, if just the image can provoke, I venture that having to *handle* an actual corpse can take fear to a new level. I have some experience to back this up.

As set by evolution's lengthy tinkering, it was the sudden surge in heart rate that alerted me I was, indeed, pretty damned scared at the prospect of laying hands on Lombardi's dead body. There's something special about the way adrenaline works. To feel your heart pound against the inside of your chest wall, with pace, is just the kind of forceful knock at the door that's required in an emergency. How clever of evolution.

One thing I'll give medical training: it forces you to face your fears. That's not to say doctors will *overcome* their fears, but exposure to what one is afraid of is generally considered the best way to extinguish anxiety. And medical training is full of the best kind of exposure—the kind you don't have a choice in.

I turned all the overheads back on (this was a task I didn't want to screw up because of dim light), walked over to the bed, and pulled the sheet down to Lombardi's waist. My hands didn't tremble outwardly as much I felt them inwardly. That was an important detail to remember for future confrontations with massive fear—they won't necessarily see you shake. Lombardi didn't look that different from a few hours earlier. I reached for his wrist, for the pulse.

His body had already started to lose its warmth. To be warm-blooded is something we all take for granted in ourselves and others; that is, until we touch a corpse. The chill of the dead startles, and reminds us by its absence that a furnace burns continuously within. It's a very disconcerting reminder. That should be enough to verify death, but the protocol has further demands.

The effort to ascertain a pulse in the newly deceased falls into the category of trying to prove a negative, which philosophers can tell you is a tougher slog. In this case, the exercise was complicated by Lombardi's anatomy coupled with my self-doubt. To feel the pulse is a matter of positioning the fingers properly. Lombardi's swollen wrist made me question *any* position as correct, and my palpitations made me wonder whether I would accidentally pick up my *own* pulse. Nevertheless, I probed a few spots as best I could, felt nothing, and moved on.

To check for spontaneous respiration was the next assessment. I had stared at Lombardi's chest as I felt for his pulse. It did not move. Just to play it safe however, I took a step back from the bed rail and got into a crouch, not as deep as a squat, but low enough that my eyes were level with the top of his convex torso. As you might see in a session of yoga, or perhaps Qigong, I held the position while my eyes locked onto the edge of his chest wall. I watched for movement and simultaneously counted my own breaths—to estimate a reasonable interval in which a living person might inhale. I was aware that certain breathing patterns produced prolonged periods of stillness, and I wanted to account for that, but finally my legs started to cramp and I stood up.

The search for heart sounds was a less ambiguous task and followed next in sequence. My stethoscope would reliably amplify Lombardi's heart valves snapping shut, if any blood flowed through them. And unlike the pulse, here I was confident of where to position my instrument. The absence of heart sounds caught me off guard, far more than the lack of pulse or respiration, and caused a little shiver. The stethoscope went back into my pocket.

I skipped the next step, responsiveness to deep pain. Why bother? Lombardi had already demonstrated a complete immunity to pain while still alive. How would that change now?

There remained one last inquiry, that of Lombardi's eyes. They were shut and would have to be manually opened to determine whether his pupils reacted to light. The principle here was not foolproof. There *were* neurologic conditions where the pupils did not react to light, but the patient was not dead. Fortunately, for physicians worried about misreading these mimics, there is another aspect of the eyes that *is* foolproof. After death, the cornea, the transparent dome that lies atop the pupil and iris, starts to turn milky, the way a windowpane frosts over. The look is unmistakable.

Opening a dead man's eyes with one's fingers seems to me at least a midlevel fear exposure exercise. A wad of thickened saliva had formed and stuck to the back of my throat. I swallowed hard, reached down, and gingerly peeled back Lombardi's lids, one at a time. The penlight then did its job. What had once been Lombardi's eyes now gave back the hazy, un-gaze of the dead. I closed them, and the redundant protocol to pronounce death was complete. He passed the test with flying colors.

Lombardi was officially dead. I looked up at the clock and noted the time: 4:23 a.m.

My heart rate had come down. After the procedure, I realized there was nothing to be afraid of. If life is sacred, surely its end deserves a careful inspection to confirm the fact.

By pure chance I had ended up Lombardi's last physician. Earlier tonight, he taught me something about what it means to be a doctor. The intimacy of the pronouncement brought me even closer to Lombardi, certainly closer than his heartless family. We were joined together in an ancient ritual—the final examination a physician performs on his patient.

I looked him over one last time, gently patted his arm, and replaced the sheet over his head.

On my way out, I turned the lights off.

POSTSCRIPT

There *were* a few more tasks I needed to complete regarding Lombardi. First, the paperwork, of course. Then there was the matter of notifying next of kin. This piqued my interest given the raw deal I felt Lombardi received. Who were these callous relations? How could they neglect basic human decency and leave their blood brother alone as he transitioned from life to death?

Not that I would interrogate them, mind you, it was not my place to judge. Nevertheless, something to their motives might be gleaned from the brief, devastating, middle-of-the-night phone call—an unwitting confession blurted amid the disorientation? I was curious.

I opened Lombardi's chart to the first page, the face sheet. It was the same in every chart—a computer-generated printout exactly 8 ½ by 11 inches in size, populated with the items deemed so vital, they should be on page one: name, date of birth, medical record number, address, phone number, emergency contact, attending physician of record, blood type, insurance carrier, insurance ID number, insurance phone number, etc.

There was a note attached to the page by a paper clip. It was for me. I removed it to take a closer look.

Handwritten by Lombardi's personal attending physician, it asked whoever pronounced Lombardi to not call the family. Instead, I was to contact him, the attending, and he would do the honors. Even better for me. This *was* a call to deliver news of death, after all. Happy to take a pass.

Now that I read the instructions, my gaze fell to the face sheet below. The portion that had been covered by the note came into focus. It was the section that listed Lombardi's diagnoses. I ran the list:

1. Congestive Heart Failure, Chronic, Severe
2. Renal Failure, Chronic, Severe
3. Alcoholic Cardiomyopathy, Chronic, Severe

Alcoholic cardiomyopathy…?

Translation: Lombardi had a disease of the heart that was a result of alcohol consumption. Alcohol is toxic to heart muscle. In alcoholic cardiomyopathy, the poisoning causes the heart to enlarge and grow weak. As the damage progresses, the pump function of the heart declines, leading to congestive heart failure. When that gets severe, renal failure can occur. Typically, this requires years and years of heavy, heavy drinking.

Oh.

ACKNOWLEDGMENTS

The stories in this collection *could* have been written without the help of the following people, but I decided to spare my readers needless suffering.

I must start by thanking my comrade in arms Dr. Rob Goldstein, a fellow psychiatrist who was also raised in Queens. It was during the collaboration on this book that Rob and I pulled up Google maps and discovered we grew up exactly one mile from each other. In Queens that's a world away, and we didn't run into each other until residency at Payne Whitney. After I realized Rob understood my stories better than I did, and was a peerless writer to boot, I asked him to be my editor. The lessons that followed—in clarity, in decorum, in pruning—dramatically improved the stories but also made me a far better writer. I am deeply grateful.

Two individuals generously gave their time to critically read large portions of manuscript. My dear neighbor Floss O'Sullivan, herself a talented writer, cast her laser focus onto many story drafts. Her questions on the material and suggestions on structure opened up possibilities hidden to me until her observations—and were immensely helpful to the final product. My sincerest thanks, Floss.

My dear wife, Bronwyn O'Neil, held somewhat captive to my process, proved herself an astute judge of continuity and punchline. Always ready for a draft with red pen and clear intuition, she could fix a struggling section with the change of a single word. Thank you Bronwyn, for your perspective and indulgence.

I want to thank the following individuals who read manuscript drafts at various stages of development and provided much appreciated encouragement: Emily Kline, Dr. Carol Weiss, Dr. Ann Beeder, Nicholas Kojak, and Deryn Mierlak.

Finally, to my team at Luminare Press, thank you for your steady hands and wise counsel.